# Terminus Brain

# Terminus Brain

## The Environmental Threats to Human Intelligence

### Christopher Williams

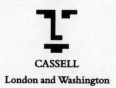

CASSELL

London and Washington

Cassell
Wellington House
125 Strand
London WC2R 0BB

PO Box 605
Herndon
VA 20172

First published 1997

**British Library Cataloguing-in-Publication Data**
A catalogue record for this book is available from the British Library.

**Library of Congress Cataloging-in-Publication Data**
Williams, Christopher.
    Terminus brain: the environmental threats to human intelligence /
Christopher Williams.
        p.    cm. — (Global issues)
    Includes bibliographical references.
    ISBN 0-304-33856-7 (hb). — ISBN 0-304-33857-5 (pb)
    1. Neurotoxicology.   2. Environmental toxicology.  3. Environmentally
induced diseases.   4. Mental handicap — Environmental aspects.   I. Title.
II. Series: Global issues
RC347.5.W54 1997
616.8′0471 — dc21

                                                                    96-29928
                                                                    CIP

ISBN 0-304-33856-7 (hardback)
        0-304-33857-5 (paperback)

Typeset by Ben Cracknell Studios
Printed and bound in Great Britain by Biddles Ltd, Guildford and King's Lynn

# Contents

# List of Figures

# Acknowledgements

Thanks to:

The Global Environmental Change programme of the UK Economic and Social Research Council (ESRC), for funding the two-year study that underpins this book, and the directors of the programme – Michael Redclift, Jim Skea and Alister Scott – for ongoing support and interest.

Dr Gwyn Prins, director, and Dee Noyes and Alison Suter, administrators at the Global Security Programme, University of Cambridge, for hosting the study, providing a way to think about the problem and daily support and encouragement.

Dr Oliver Russell, Director of the Norah Fry Research Centre, University of Bristol, for encouragement and help during the initial planning of the project, and for providing the opportunity to learn from and about the people whom the study concerns.

Sheena Mackenzie, information officer at the Norah Fry Research Centre, and the Scottish Office Education and Industry Department, for initial data searches, readings of drafts and insightful discussion, design work and very much else.

Merlin Willcox, Keble College, Oxford, Dr Lynne Jones, Cambridge, and Lesley Millner, for providing valuable comments on parts of the draft manuscript.

Trockel Ulmann & Freunde, one of the few cafes in Cambridge that has not become part of the academic theme park, for providing endless coffee, friendship and sanctuary while I was reading, thinking and correcting drafts.

The many, including people labelled as having intellectual disabilities, in the UK, India, China, Thailand, Turkey, the USA and elsewhere, for unknowingly contributing through a comment, thought or story, or just by being themselves.

The staff at Cassell – Jane Greenwood, Sandra Margolies and Libby Ridgeway – for encouragement, constructive help and the inevitable but invisible work that ultimately turns a manuscript into a book.

As always, final responsibility for error and opinion rests with the author, who would be grateful to receive constructive comments about factual inaccuracies.

# PART I

# The Threat to Intelligence

# CHAPTER 1

# Terminus Brain

The human brain is now at risk from itself. Like a terminus, it is an end-point of our environmental mistakes, but it is also the starting-point of those mistakes and of their correction. It is victim, perpetrator and healer of adverse environmental change, which we now know can impair intellectual functioning.

Our intelligence – how we know, how we reason, how we learn – is how we survive. For individuals, most brain impairment is irreversible, so the personal cost is obvious and often drastic, and the nature of the injury inherently diminishes the ability of those who suffer to counter the cause. For communities, the consequences of widespread intellectual decline are simple to envisage but hard to detect, so our collective response to this particular environmental threat is also minimal.

For millions of years our brain has enjoyed a positive interaction with its environment, which has given rise to progressive brain development. Now this could alter. In the long history of human evolution, the brain's current threat to itself is a novel situation, and this gives rise to the possibility of regressive brain evolution in specific communities. Our brain is the only thing in the ecosystem that directly jeopardizes its own well-being, which suggests a unique form of ecological vulnerability.

The human brain should logically be a priority of environmental concern, but it is not. How and why is Terminus Brain now at risk from its own behaviour, and what does this mean for individual and human survival?

Throughout the world, up to 3 per cent of any community are considered to have an intellectual disability, defined in Western clinical terms such as 'mental handicap', or acknowledged in more traditional understandings like the African Shona *dununu*, but in some regions levels now approach 20 per cent. This is often paralleled by a much greater incidence of milder, 'sub-clinical' intellectual dysfunction. In some African cities more than 90 per cent of children now have blood lead levels that can cause intellectual problems.

The reason is the *presence* of environmental agents that destroy intellectual potential, such as heavy metals or radiation, and the *absence* of environmental macro- and micro-nutrients necessary for the proper development and functioning of the brain, such as iodine or iron. There are also adverse *synergisms* between the two, which appear significant but are usually missed from standard analysis. Iron deficiency can precipitate the body's uptake of lead, for instance.

Assessment of the environmental threat to human intelligence is uniquely difficult, not least because there is no single word to describe it. The starting-point is therefore to use a collective term: environmentally-mediated intellectual decline or EMID. Despite inadequate conceptualization, there is now enough evidence to demonstrate significant problems on a small scale. The question *Terminus Brain* asks is therefore straightforward: are the existing small-scale instances of EMID indicative of something bigger?

---

Impacts on the brain are described by many different and overlapping terms – none specifically indicating environmental causation. Throughout this book, when discussion derives from specific sources, the terminology of the source has been preserved. In general:

- *intellectual disability* relates to the more serious, permanent impairments bearing labels such as 'mental handicap', 'mental retardation', 'learning disabilities' – often called *clinical* outcomes;
- *intellectual dysfunction* describes the numerous less serious permanent or temporary conditions, such as reduced perception, learning ability, memory or cognitive functions – often called *subclinical* outcomes;
- *intellectual decline* embraces both.

The overall circumstance is called environmentally-mediated intellectual decline:

- 'mediated' to stress that human act or omission and not 'the environment' is the root cause of the problem;
- 'decline' describing the effect on the intellectual potential of individuals and populations.

Environmentally-mediated intellectual decline is abbreviated as EMID.

---

The effects of our environmental mistakes take numerous forms. Many are rendered harmless by biological eco-mechanisms. Some enter the human food chain and others act on the human body through inhalation, or skin or sensory penetration, perhaps then affecting the blood, body tissue or genes. The routes are complex and countless, and the human brain is an end-point.

In Buckminster Fuller's words, 'the body is the mobile environment of the brain', and it is a special environment which provides a battery of defences against toxic attack on the brain: the liver, kidney and, more specifically, the blood–brain barrier and the nose–brain barrier. From the human perspective, the routes of environmental threats, within ecological and bodily environments, might also be viewed as the natural defences protecting the major terminus – human intelligence.

But this is a human-centred view. From an ecological perspective the human brain is not the terminus, just another station on a circular line: a station that can be closed down and by-passed if it does not serve to benefit the whole system. If human intelligence is a specific threat to the survival of an ecosystem, then that system might protect itself by curtailing the destructive capabilities of that intelligence. A population with a maximum IQ of 70 would not threaten the ecosystem through running nuclear power stations, creating toxic pollutants or manufacturing cars. Perhaps the vision seems utopian – but a visit to the dentist would not be much fun. So *Terminus Brain* assumes a human viewpoint – that we wish to remain part of the ecosystem, and in a positive human condition above that of bare biological survival.

Visions of an environmentally mediated end to human populations are usually portrayed in life-or-death terms, stemming from the Malthusian view that increasing numbers will be curtailed by finite resources. But such clear-cut prognoses omit a significant intermediate stage before widespread death: a period during which there would be a general reduction of human capacity. Malnutrition, micro-nutrient deficiency and pollution would bring about a gradual decline in intellectual and related functioning. The growing environmental threat is less a matter of life or death, and more one of life or half-life for millions of our global family.

Intellectual disability is a natural part of human existence and, as individuals, those who have intellectual disabilities clearly enrich the meaning of that existence. But unnaturally high numbers combined with a hidden level of 'sub-clinical' decline, caused by EMID, pose problems for any community.

The linkages between national development, human survival and intellectual potential are usually confined to discussion of the improvement of human resources through education. Much less policy consideration has been given to the other side of the equation, the biological *potential* to learn, which can be reduced by external factors in our chemical, physical and human environment. There is great concern about children who *do not*, from a pedagogical perspective, learn. But concern about the increasing numbers of those who, because of adverse environmental change, *cannot* learn effectively usually falls outside the mainstream education and development debate. Literacy statistics, for instance, do not distinguish between those who are illiterate because they have not had the chance to learn to read and write, and those who have had the opportunity but do not have the intellectual ability to learn.

This one-sided view of intellectual resources, which still underpins our global educational policy, is put into a broader perspective by James Lovelock:

> *Human brains . . . did not develop as a result of the natural selective advantage of passing examinations, nor indeed so that we could perform any of the feats of memory and other mental exercises now explicitly required for education.*[1]

Educational and social influences are very important, probably more important than is generally accepted, but the *primary* factors influencing the potential of the brain are biological. No form of education or social intervention can mend damaged brain cells.

The intellectual potential of individuals and communities must be maintained in optimum condition to achieve positive survival. An awakening concern within scientific communities, international agencies and the US government suggests that this should become a crucial environmental priority of the future. But will it? This chapter concludes with a reminder of the distinctive nature of the politics of EMID, which may stop this happening.

## An awakening concern: the 'Decade of the Brain'

Nineteen eighty-nine was the year in which the US government could start to turn its mind from the old security threats of the Cold War towards the new 'threats without enemies' in the form of escalating environmental problems.[2] In that year, in the wake of a growing concern about environmental neurotoxins from academics and environmental pressure groups, the 101st US Congress declared the 1990s the Decade of the Brain.[3]

The Neurotoxicology Division of the Environmental Protection Agency (EPA) in North Carolina became the largest neurotoxicology group in the world, with a capacity to work across a broad spectrum of relevant science from the molecular to the behavioural level. In the following year, the Congress Office of Technology Assessment (OTA) produced a key report, *Neurotoxicity: Identifying and Controlling Poisons of the Nervous System*.[4] This developed the realization that environmental medicine had for too long concentrated on cancer as the main outcome of human-caused environmental change, while ignoring the perhaps more important effects on the human brain.[5] Detecting cancer is reasonably straightforward because it is clinically visible. Effects on intelligence are very difficult to establish because the outcomes are multifaceted and represent a continuum with no clear cut-off point.

Before 1990, related interest within the US government was confined to the 'bounded', and politically less sensitive, environments of home and work – *Neurotoxins at Home and in the Workplace* stemmed from hearings before a Congress sub-committee in 1986.[6] Neuro-degenerative disease associated with ageing was discussed in a brief background paper in 1984, *Impacts of Neuroscience*,[7] and the following years saw an increasing belief that this might, in part, be linked to environmental toxins such as aluminium.

Another Congress report, *The Nature and Extent of Lead Poisoning in Children in the United States*, tackled once again the politically more sensitive question of environmental lead.[8] From the US Centers for Disease Control and Prevention came *Preventing Lead Poisoning in Young Children*[9] in 1991, which called for a further lowering of the 'safe level' for blood lead and for universal screening of children. This marked the start of a major campaign by the US government to reduce lead exposure. The US National Academy of Sciences produced a report, *Measuring Lead Exposure in Infants, Children and Other Sensitive Populations*, which made similar points and formally concluded that some people in any population are more vulnerable to environmental threats to the brain.[10]

The general concern was then taken up by the US National Research Council in 1992, which marked a new medical discipline in the title of the book *Environmental Neurotoxicology*. This, for the first time, put the brain as a focus for environmental medicine, challenging scientists to find out if the visible signs and symptoms diagnosable by clinical means, and the effects of recognized industrial disasters, are just the tip of a largely sub-clinical and creeping-disaster iceberg.

> A major unanswered question – indeed, a central issue confronting neurotoxicology today – is whether the causal associations observed in epidemics of neurotoxic diseases reflect isolated events or are merely the most obvious examples of a widespread association between environmental chemicals and nervous system impairment.[11]

A review of *Environmental Neurotoxicology* in the journal *Science*, 'Zeroing in on brain toxins', reiterated a key issue raised by the report: the previous emphasis on cancer at the expense of assessing the environmental effects on the brain.[12] It also remarked on the authors' iconoclastic lack of faith in some of the traditional scientific techniques used in risk assessment, when applied to the brain.

At the same time, the US government started to investigate more specific, and commercially sensitive, issues such as neurotoxic pesticides and the farmworker.[13] The effects of substance abuse were brought into focus in *Drugs and the Brain*[14] and *Assessing Neurotoxicity of Drugs Abuse*.[15] The outcome of this governmental interest was a range of books from the US medical community, of which *The Vulnerable Brain and Environmental Risks* is typical.[16] In 1996, a group of international scientists marked a growing concern about a newer form of threat from the synthetic hormone-disrupting chemicals, which appears potentially more problematic even than lead, in the Erice Statement (see Appendix).

The concern within the USA, based mainly on toxicology, is largely related to the effects of the *presence* of hazardous environmental agents – 'the environmental problem' from a rich-nation, urbanized perspective. This is only half the picture. During the 1990s, UNICEF and the World Health Organization (WHO) were increasing their campaigns to redress the *absence* of environmental agents necessary for proper human development – micro-nutrient deficiency or 'hidden hunger' – which has only very recently been conceptualized as an environmental problem associated with land degradation and deforestation. In 1996, *Scientific American* reported new understandings about the relationships between malnutrition, poverty and intellectual development.[17] *New Scientist* affirmed the link between micro-nutrient deficiencies and intellectual decline caused by the Green Revolution.[18] Protein–energy malnutrition (PEM), for example, now dulls the minds of millions of children in poorer countries.

A specific concern of UNICEF and WHO is iodine deficiency, a major threat to the human brain lucidly explained by Basil Hetzel in *The Story of Iodine Deficiency*[19] and *SOS for a Billion: The Conquest of Iodine Deficiency Disorders*.[20] Hence came the establishment of the International Council for Control of Iodine Deficiency (ICCID), and research centres such as the Program against Micronutrient Malnutrition (PAMM) at Emory University, Atlanta, which also deals with other micro-nutrient problems. In 1990, the UN World Health Assembly endorsed a Global Action Plan on iodine deficiency, put forward by the ICCID.

So the Decade of the Brain has seen these two parallel environmental perspectives – problems caused by the *presence* and by the *absence* of environmental agents. But because these two aspects broadly reflect the urban/pollution/rich-world versus rural/malnutrition/poor-world stereotypes, they have not been viewed together. As the world globalizes at an increasing rate, such polarized perspectives are fast becoming meaningless frames of reference for millions of people.

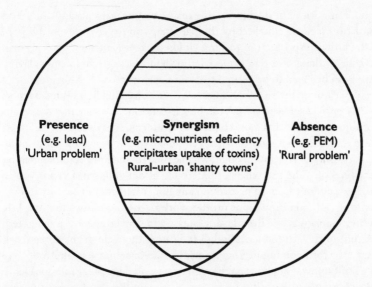

**Figure 1.1** The EMID paradigm.

A comprehensive understanding is crucial, not least because the research needed to address the problem is largely dictated by rich-nation priorities and this must be questioned – the US Decade of the Brain relates to only a part of the global problem. The dissipated nature of the relevant medical disciplines, muddled terminology and diverse and inconsistent regional policy create many different islands of specialist understanding, which further obscure an effective overview.

The main purpose of *Terminus Brain* is therefore to create a framework for a comprehensive understanding. The overall paradigm is *presence*-EMID, *absence*-EMID and synergistic effects between the two. This paradigm is both biological and social. For example, the world's burgeoning 'shanty towns' create the social context where the 'rural' malnutrition and 'urban' pollution threats come together and compound one another (Figure 1.1).

## The politics of EMID: hype and denial

In the wake of discussing any new concern there is, of course, the danger of creating emotive scare stories. 'Children and brain damage' have been the ingredients of countless media hypes. British 'mad cow disease' (BSE/CJD) in 1996 is but one example. Medical reputations can be made on the basis of research concerning a dozen subjects, which is then expressed as percentages, giving the impression of a globally applicable generalization. Hype can be compounded through an understandable desire by parents of children born with disabilities to explain, and perhaps place blame. The situation is further fuelled by the parental wish to have clever children, which finds expression in feeding children excessive amounts of sugar in Russia or the increase in piano sales in Beijing – sugar and piano-playing are both believed to be related to brain development.

Conclusions, such as one from the UK National Children's Bureau report *Children and the Environment*,[21] can be self-defeating. To state that the results of a study 'suggest that most children in British cities have absorbed enough lead to hinder their intellectual development' may be arguable in scientific circles. But the conclusion could well be used to underpin comments along the lines of, 'Then so what? Look around at our children. Even if you're right, it doesn't seem to be making any noticeable difference.' In 1996, a cost of £10 billion was put on the work needed to ensure that the UK water supply was free from lead. Doubtless the government was delighted. A sum of this magnitude, though indicating the scale of the threat, will never be forthcoming, so the problem could once more be shelved.

The timing of public-awareness exercises is also delicate. Professor Derek Bryce-Smith of Reading University has been the key figure in raising concern about lead in petrol in the UK since the 1950s. Subsequent science has proved his general assertions to be correct, and his conclusions have informed government policy about lead in many countries. During the Scarman inquiry into the Brixton riots (London), he argued that behavioural problems arising from high lead levels were an underlying cause of the disturbances. The evidence linking lead with behaviour problems is now rarely disputed, and it may appear self-evident that such riots are therefore more probable in a community suffering lead poisoning. But these arguments were politically inappropriate so close to an emotive event, and the reputation of Bryce-Smith suffered as a result.

It is also interesting to note situations that *are* made highly visible by governments. From China, the figure of eight million people suffering iodine deficiency-related intellectual disability results from official research and is widely quoted by state sources.[22] Yet in the same country, when car ownership triples in three years and unleaded petrol is not available, these circumstances will certainly create levels of intellectual decline that will equate with the levels caused by iodine deficiency. The world is not told about this problem by the Chinese government. Iodine deficiency does not obviously result from poor political management; bad transport planning does. National programmes to remedy iodine deficiency attract foreign currency in the form of aid and have no negative consequences; attempts to reduce car pollution might affect the perception of the exploding consumer economy which the government believes will prevent further expressions of public discontent like that at Tiananmen Square.

It is very proper that governments should not precipitate or fuel scare stories that could disrupt necessary economic development, or cause unnecessary fear. But due caution must be balanced with an awareness of the dynamics that lead to a denial of this particular problem. The US A-bombs dropped on Nagasaki and Hiroshima propagated many myths about 'brain damage' and 'genetic mutation', which had been dismissed by scientists and governments for decades. But the year 1990 saw another, little-noticed, publication from the US National Research Council, *Health Effects of Exposure to Low Levels of Ionizing Radiation*. Data were finally made available indicating 'a major (and dose–response related) increase in severe mental retardation', together with sub-clinical effects on school performance, among survivors of the A-bomb.[23] Why did we need to wait until the survivors were 45 years of age to learn that they were severely mentally retarded (which is evident by the age of 2) and to be able to assess their school performance? Is it a coincidence that these data, which may well have fuelled anti-nuclear protest from a very emotive human standpoint, did not become public until the Cold War had ended?

The political desire to control discussion is universal. The Soviet nuclear industry disaster at Chernobyl provides the classic example. Reports from scientists and doctors about an increase in genetic abnormalities in animals and human infants were initially dismissed by the Soviet establishment as 'statistically insignificant blips'. In 1986, the Ministry of Public Health issued a gagging order.[24] Discussing the risk of intellectual decline, Ivan Holowinsky concludes:

> *Efforts to assess the extent of the catastrophe have been obstructed by the Soviets, who have been reluctant to discuss the effects of radiation on newborns and children. This secretive attitude directly prevents the possibility of the accurate assessment of the incidence of mental retardation that can be attributed to this nuclear explosion.*[25]

But communist attitudes were not the only impediment to assessment. In 1991, WHO planned to support a project to assess 'brain damage *in utero*', but later in the year funds were frozen without explanation.

Radiation was not the only threat to be covered up during the Cold War. Mercury leaks (2.4 million pounds 'lost') from the Union Carbide Y-12 weapons installation at Oak Ridge, Tennessee, caused the highest ever recorded levels of mercury pollution in local rivers, yet local people were not warned of dangerous levels in fish because the reports were classified information. A later Congressional investigation concluded that classification 'provided a convenient shield behind which the nonsensitive but politically volatile data on the quantity of mercury releases could be buried and obscured'.[26]

11

Even after the fall of the Berlin Wall, in 1990, the KGB forbade Dr Kaydyrbek Andagulov from diagnosing lead poisoning following an unplanned release from the Oskemen smelter, which produced nearly half of the USSR's zinc and lead. Further secret monitoring found that the whole population had hazardous body burdens of lead.[27] Obfuscation in relation to military endeavour is not just a prerogative of communist regimes. The 1985 Evatt Royal Commission, in Australia, stated that exposure of civilians to Agent Orange had little or no effect on birth abnormalities. This was later challenged because such conclusions could not have been drawn from the evidence available to the inquiry.[28]

If the Cold War were the only reason for control of information, the problem of denial might need little further discussion, but this is not the case. Environmental activists in India, who draw attention to the worrying levels of intellectual and other disabilities around the nuclear power stations in Rajasthan, do so at risk of committing an offence. It is unlawful to discuss nuclear power stations, ostensibly because of military implications.

Military security may explain, and perhaps even excuse, some cover-ups. But in other spheres the reason is more mundane – money. Damages awards to individuals, relating to brain injury (usually in relation to medical negligence), between 1992 and 1994 in the British Isles ranged between £1.5 and £7 million. If we start to view EMID in justice terms for whole populations, it could cost the responsible entities dearly, and it is therefore not difficult to see why there may be a motivation to manage public perception of the problem. The cash consequences of admitting a link between industrial poisoning and brain injury are usually so massive that the money made available to refute links is virtually limitless.

Political obfuscation can be linked to commercial interests. Robin Russell questions why, in the UK, the 1994 House of Commons Transport Committee's report on air pollution in London 'called for a ban on the sale of superunleaded petrol and criticized the use of premium unleaded fuel in cars not fitted with catalytic converters . . . [yet] the committee did not invite any evidence on the adverse health effects of lead', and accepted uncritically 'evidence submitted to their inquiry by Associated Octel, Britain's sole manufacturer of lead additives for petrol'.[29] It is interesting to note the omissions in the key US Congress report *Neurotoxicity*: nicotine and alcohol, which have commercial ramifications; and radioactive chemicals and biological and chemical warfare, which have military implications.[30]

More overt forms of information management by commercial interests are reported in relation to health monitoring of young women in the *maquiladora* factories on the Mexico–USA border, where there is widespread concern about the level of physical and mental impairments in young children. Potential mothers employed in hazardous jobs are routinely sacked after working for short periods. This creates an impression of a healthy workforce and, because the women have worked in numerous locations, any health problems cannot be attributed to one particular factory. Epidemiological studies have mixed high- and low-risk groups, which weakens the data, and the follow-up period of studies is often too short, so time-latent outcomes are omitted. Similar circumstances surrounded the UK-based firm Thor Chemicals. At its factory in South Africa workers were exposed to high levels of mercury, which were linked to death and neurological disorders. Casual workers were reportedly employed for the more hazardous jobs, and they were dismissed when neurological symptoms appeared.

The nuclear industry is particularly sensitive and particularly powerful. In 1994, Greenpeace UK ran an advertisement showing a child with hydrocephalus (a form of brain injury creating an enlarged head), which was labelled 'Kazakhstan nuclear test victim'. Following immediate complaints from the British nuclear industry, the Advertising Standards Authority censured Greenpeace, saying that the link between radiation and hydrocephalus was unproven and there was no proof that the child featured was a nuclear test victim. Whoever is in the right, the interesting aspect is this reaction by the nuclear industry. Had the same picture appeared in another guise during the Cold War era, it might have been taken as patriotic propaganda against the Soviets.

Political and commercial obfuscation is compounded at other levels in a community. The social and personal outcomes of intellectual disability unfortunately, but often inevitably, lead to a desire for secrecy. There is an understandable reluctance to fuel stories of intellectual decline in Indian or Chinese villages in which the possibility of offspring being born with disability may spoil marriage opportunities. This wish to hide the problem is not unreasonable at local levels. But the medical world often then acquiesces to the social desire to hide away people with intellectual disabilities by hospitalizing those who could very well exist within a community. At one institution in India it was reported how

> wardens and janitors took bribes to facilitate admissions . . . Families often
> deliver new patients to the hospital in chains . . . Nearly 300 patients at
> Ranchi have been declared 'socially cured' and could return home, but their
> families won't take them.[31]

Thomas Midgley invented chlorofluorocarbons (CFCs) *and* put lead into petrol. The link between ozone depletion and CFCs has been argued for only a few years; the link between lead and human health has been recognized for two millennia. Both can be conceptualized as global environmental problems. Like the profile of CFC use, we know, for example, that Africa contributes 20 per cent of atmospheric lead pollution and that North America's output has reduced significantly. Yet lead has not been presented to the public as a 'global environmental problem'. Recent action concerning CFCs has been swift and international, as compared to a few isolated national initiatives to reduce, but not eliminate, environmental lead.

The desire to deny EMID can therefore exist at *all* levels of society. States, local communities and families fail individuals, who because of the nature of their injury are unlikely to put their case. Vested commercial interests lead to further obfuscation, and over-enthusiastic advocacy or hype can be counterproductive. There seems little likelihood that EMID will ever be high on the environmental agenda – there are probably more eco-votes in saving whales, preventing cancer or reversing sperm demise than in protecting brain cells. The medical profession is primarily concerned with cures. There is no cure for intellectual disability, so clinical interest is sidelined, creating a Cinderella subject within medicine pursued only by a visionary minority. These dynamics are a distinctive aspect of EMID. Who will take up the case on behalf of individuals and communities who are, or might be, affected? Who has the responsibility to assess what is happening and protect our global intellectual resources? Who or what will protect our brain from itself?

The first problem of assessing the impact of EMID is to obtain reliable statistics. Chapter 2 brings together the available evidence, and reminds us why data are so difficult to come by. But figures are only one aspect. The individual and social cost consequences provide the other important arguments.

The rest of the book is framed within the four relevant 'environments' of the problem – the human body, the social, the ecological and the conceptual (Figure 1.2).

Chapter 3 outlines the necessary medical understandings, but emphasizes how little we know. These limits of knowledge become more apparent when viewed over a time frame, as in Chapter 4. The faith that we have in 'risk assessment' is misguided. This is in part because standard procedures do not work well when the brain is the end-point of environmental threats, but also because the basis upon which calculations are founded reflects scientific convenience rather than the global human rights consensus – that we should aim to protect the most vulnerable, not simply ensure the survival of the fittest.

We cannot change human biology or the fundamental way in which environmental chemicals react with one another, but we can encourage changes in human behaviour. Chapters 5, 6 and 7 therefore develop social understandings within the 'bounded' environments of home and workplace,

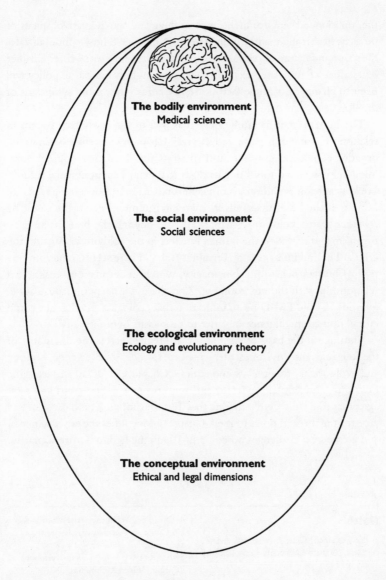

**Figure 1.2**   The four environments of the brain.

the 'unbounded' environment beyond these and the 'pervasive' spirals of poverty, health and malnutrition. The main message is how politics dictates the scope and nature of relevant research. Can we find a social cure? Chapter 8 describes a few isolated examples, and suggests how education policy will need to change. But these factors are not cures – just more symptoms of the ill.

The human brain is rarely viewed as part of the ecosystem system in relation to its and our continued survival. Chapter 9 therefore outlines the broader ecological context, and suggests the need to recognize how 'modernity super-vectors' bring us closer to potential environmental hazards. Looking at brain evolution over millennia raises a more concerning scenario. Now that the brain threatens its own environment, could the result be *regressive* brain evolution? Chapter 10 goes beyond the brain as an eco-organism and considers the human intellect in the ecosystem. What of the outward bound influences of Terminus Brain? There seems to be a unique trait of human behaviour, pertinacity, which underpins our conflictual relationship with the environment. And there is a deeper, if speculative, question. Could EMID be an indication that ecological intelligence could curtail human intelligence in order to protect its own interests?

Arguing on the basis of current inconsistencies across the disciplines of the four relevant 'environments' – medical science, social science, ecology and evolutionary theory, law and ethics – Chapters 11, 12 and 13 examine how our 'conceptual environment' requires new perceptions and new agreements. Finally, remembering that Terminus Brain is both cause of and cure for the threat it poses to itself, Chapter 14 identifies the environmental and intellectual challenges posed by EMID in the light of future scenarios.

## Notes

1. J.E. Lovelock, *Gaia: A New Look at Life on Earth*, (Oxford University Press: Oxford 1979), p. 149.

2. Gwyn Prins (ed.), *Threats without Enemies: Facing Environmental Insecurity* (Earthscan Publications: London, 1993).

3. US Congress, *The Decade of the Brain – Public Law 101–58* (US Government Printing Office: Washington, DC, 1989).

4. Office of Technology Assessment, US Congress, *Neurotoxicity: Identifying and Controlling Poisons of the Nervous System*, OTA-BA-436 (US Government Printing Office: Washington, DC, 1990).

5. Federal Focus, *Toward Common Measures: Recommendations for a Presidential Executive Order on Environmental Risk Assessment and Risk Management Policy* (Federal Focus: Washington, DC, 1991), pp. 66–9.

6. US Congress, *Neurotoxins at Home and in the Workplace: Report* (Y1.1/8:99-827, 87-3985, 90.7266) (US Congress, House Committee on Science and Technology: Washington, DC, 1990).

7. US Congress/OTA, *Impacts of Neuroscience – Background Paper*, OTA-BP-BA-24 (US Government Printing Office: Washington, DC, 1984).

8. ATSDR (US Dept HHS), *The Nature and Extent of Lead Poisoning in Children in the United States* (US Congress: Atlanta, GA, 1991).

9. Centers for Disease Control and Prevention, *Preventing Lead Poisoning in Young Children* (US Government Printing Office: Washington, DC, 1991).

10. National Academy of Sciences, *Measuring Lead Exposure in Infants, Children and Other Sensitive Populations* (National Academy of Sciences: Washington, DC, 1993).

11. National Research Council, *Environmental Neurotoxicology* (National Academy Press: Washington, DC, 1992), p. 2.

12. Richard Stone, 'Zeroing in on brain toxins', *Science* (1992), **255**, 1063.

13. Ellen Widness, *Neurotoxic Pesticides and the Farmworker: A Report* (Y3.T 22/2:2N 39/2/neurot) 92-8672 (US Government Printing Office: Washington, DC, 1992).

14. David P. Friedman, *Drugs and the Brain* (HE 20.3031:D 84/993) 94-4608 (US Government Printing Office: Washington, DC, 1994).

15. US Congress, *Assessing Neurotoxicity of Drugs Abuse* (HE 20.828216:136) 94-4650 (US Government Printing Office: Washington, DC, 1994).

16. Robert L. Isaacson and Karl Jenson (eds), *The Vulnerable Brain and Environmental Risks* (Plenum: London, 1994).

17. L.J. Brown and E. Pollitt, 'Malnutrition, poverty and intellectual development', *Scientific American* (1996), **274** (2), 26–31.

18. Jane Seymour, 'Hungry for a new revolution', *New Scientist* (1996), **2023**, 32–7.

19. Basil S. Hetzel, *The Story of Iodine Deficiency: An International Challenge in Nutrition* (Oxford University Press: Oxford, 1989).

20. B.S. Hetzel and C.S. Pandav, *SOS for a Billion: The Conquest of Iodine Deficiency Disorders* (Oxford University Press: Oxford, 1994).

21. Martin Rosenbaum, *Children and the Environment* (National Children's Bureau: London, 1993), p. 9.

22. Richard Tomlinson, 'Eight million Chinese with reduced IQ because of iodine shortage', *British Medical Journal* (1995), **310**, 146.

23. NRC, *Health Effects of Exposure to Low Levels of Ionizing Radiation* (BEIR V) (National Academy Press: Washington, DC, 1990).

24. Murray Feshbach and Alfred Friendly, *Ecocide in the USSR* (Aurum Press: London, 1992), p. 152.

25. Ivan Z. Holowinsky, 'Chernobyl nuclear catastrophe and the high risk potential for mental retardation', *Mental Retardation* (1993), **31**(1), 35–40.

26. D. Dembo, W. Morehouse and L. Wyhle, *Abuse of Power* (New Horizons Press: New York, 1993).

27. Mike Edwards, 'Lethal legacy', *National Geographic* (1994), **186** (2), 92.

28. 'Update . . . Agent Orange', *Pacific Research* (1990), **3**(1), 20.

29. Robin Russell, 'A time bomb in your tank?' *Guardian*, 9 November 1994, p. 2.

30. Office of Technology Assessment, US Congress, *Neurotoxicity: Identifying and Controlling Poisons of the Nervous System*, OTA-BA-436 (US Government Printing Office: Washington, DC, 1990), p. 4.

31. Christopher Williams, *The Right to Be Known: A Global View of Human Rights and Mental Handicap* (Norah Fry Research Centre, University of Bristol: Bristol, 1993), p. 34.

# CHAPTER 2

# Why the Concern?

Why the concern – why *now* a sudden concern? The environmental threat to human intelligence is not entirely new. The first part of the answer comes from an awareness of the scale of the problem and of the difficulties in achieving reliable statistics. But figures do not tell the whole story. It is equally important to envisage the personal and social costs and consequences of environmentally-mediated intellectual decline. Whatever the scale, the human outcome cannot be dismissed lightly. There are no convenient global figures or simple sound bites. Like a jigsaw, the overall picture becomes clear only when many apparently unrelated pieces are put into place.

## Scale of effect

Intellectual decline is more a social construct than a medical condition, and environmental threats are ill-defined. With both outcome and cause so intangible, it is unsurprising that statistics indicating a level of EMID are scarce and imprecise. The US National Research Council concludes:

> *The number of people with neurotoxic disorders and the extent of neurologic disease and dysfunction that result from exposure to toxic chemicals in the environment are not known . . . The data needed to estimate the overall magnitude of the problem of environmental neurotoxicity do not exist.*[1]

And this is in state-of-the-art America, and only relates to half the problem – *presence*-EMID.

Two general considerations provide a starting-point for gaining a comprehensive impression of scale. First, the causes of many intellectual disabilities are unknown. One Western expert concludes, 'At least a third of cases do not have any obvious aetiology . . . Clearly, mental retardation . . . has a complex basis that includes monogenic and polygenic disorders, chromosomal abnormalities, and a number of ill-defined environmental factors.'[2] In non-Western settings this can be even higher. In Bahrain the figure is 42 per cent of cases with an 'untraceable' cause.[3]

The second task is to consider health and the environment as an indicator of EMID. In 1989, the Supreme Soviet Environmental Committee reported that '80% of the diseases in the USSR relate, directly or indirectly, to environmental problems'.[4] It is not unreasonable to infer a significant level of intellectual decline within a population with this magnitude of environmental health problems.

The people of Kara-Kalpakskaya, situated around the southern end of the ill-fated Aral Sea, are reported to be 'dying like flies' because of environmental conditions. There are high levels of heavy metals and other toxins in water supplies; food is still being contaminated by pesticides such as DDT; the area is blighted by radiation from bomb testing. In ten years, kidney and liver diseases have increased up to 40-fold, which reduces the body's biological defences against neurotoxins. Many women have high levels of lead, zinc and strontium in their blood and 23 per cent suffer thyroid dysfunctions. The area has the highest level of infant mortality in the former Soviet Union. North of the Aral, 99 per cent of pregnant women are anaemic, as are most children. Iron-deficiency anaemia is a major cause of sub-clinical intellectual decline.

Data concerning lead provide the most common source demonstrating *presence*-EMID. It is now officially accepted that one-sixth of the children in the USA 'have an excessive lead body burden that impairs health and interferes with the ability to learn'; in California, it is one-fifth. Because of the blood lead levels in potential mothers in the USA, it is projected that these women 'may be expected to bear some 10 million children at risk of lead poisoning at birth'.[5] General statistics sometimes hide acute situations in particular communities. It was found that in Bunker Hill, Idaho, 'all children tested had high-level lead poisoning'.[6] In 1993, France suddenly discovered that 10 per cent of a sample of poor Parisian children suffered lead poisoning and that 'thousands were threatened with irreversible neurological lesions'.[7] Bear in mind that all this is in rich nations where protection standards are relatively high.

Unsurprisingly, the situation in poorer communities is sometimes much worse. Jerome Nriagu of the University of Michigan found that by applying American standards, 'more than 90 per cent of children in some African cities suffer from lead poisoning'.[8] In Mexico City 'one quarter of all babies are born with enough lead in their blood permanently to damage their brains'.[9] A study of Managuan children exposed to lead through industrial processes, by the Dutch epidemiologist Françoise Barten, found that, in the urban area of high exposure, 60 per cent had levels exceeding the US federal definition of lead toxicity (100 micrograms of lead per litre of blood) which is linked with decreased mental development. Within a rural control group, not suffering direct exposure, no children exceeded this level.[11] The

> Reliable statistical information rarely exists in the former USSR, but scattered sources evidence a link between general pollution and intellectual disability.
>
> Congenitally deformed children were being born in the Soviet capital 'one and a half times more often' on average than in the USSR as a whole.
>
> In one heavily polluted district of [Kemerovo], retardation among children was 2.1 times more frequent than in a cleaner neighbourhood on the opposite bank of the Tom river.
>
> The Kemerovo statistic on child retardation echoed a national one: From 1975 to 1990 the rate at which women gave birth to retarded children – nearly 2 million by 1991 – increased more than twice as fast in the USSR's big cities as in the countryside.
>
> In the 1980s congenital deformities, mostly retardation, appeared among children born to twenty-six of the town's five hundred families. 'We found a link', wrote Dr Airiyan, who worked in the Ararat Valley since 1953, 'between the extensive use of poisonous chemicals [in agriculture] . . . and the rise in congenital diseases.'
>
> The doctor found that the Moldovan . . . children, many of them mentally handicapped, were 30 to 40 percent behind their healthier contemporaries in physical development.
>
> . . . in Magnitogorsk . . . birth defects in the city have doubled since 1980 . . . not only was infant mortality high . . . but one-fourth of all the infants who died were born with congenital development defects.
>
> From 1988 to 1990 in Yaroslavl, also the site of a major lead-processing factory . . . and other large polluting enterprises . . . rates of congenital abnormalities among children quadrupled.[10]

World Bank has identified 37 'hot spots' – within Poland, the Czech Republic, Hungary, Bulgaria, Romania, Russia and Ukraine – where lead threatens children's intellectual development.[12]

Looking beyond lead, a landmark study of the effects of congenital poisoning by polychlorinated biphenyls (PCBs) in Taiwan found that 10 per cent of exposed children suffered psychomotor delay and 7 per cent speech problems, compared to 3 per cent among control groups.[13] This represents a doubling and tripling of children with difficulties, just from a single pollutant. Colborn *et al.* warn in *Our Stolen Future* of the problems created by these new chemicals. Five per cent of US babies are now exposed to PCBs in breast milk to a degree that could affect their neurological development.[14]

Statistics are sometimes presented in a more innovative way, which can illuminate the formal prevalence figures. Geordie Greig, reporting the alarming increase in intellectual disability in children born to mothers who use crack cocaine in the USA, points out that 'every 90 seconds a baby is born suffering from exposure to cocaine. Last year [1991], 375,000 babies were infected in the womb by one or more illicit drugs.'[15] Intellectual decline in old age is another part of the picture. Alzheimer's disease, which may in part be linked to environmental toxins such as aluminium, affects one person in 1000 aged between 40 and 65.

'Hidden hunger' – micro-nutrient deficiencies which cause much of *absence*-EMID – is reckoned now to affect more than two billion people throughout the world.[16] Intellectual decline caused by iodine deficiency disorders (IDDs) provides the most readily available source of statistics, because causation is easy to establish clinically, and it is politically unproblematic. The UNICEF 1994 *Annual Report* warned that, in addition to the serious and recognizable outcome, cretinism, 'the intellectual capacity of entire populations may be reduced by up to 10 per cent'.[17] UNICEF estimates that 1.6 billion people live in areas where dietary intake of iodine is inadequate (30 per cent of the world's population); 655 million people have affected thyroid glands and an 'increasing risk of mental impairment'; 26 million suffer brain damage; 5.7 million suffer cretinism, the most severe form of the disorder. A total of 300 million people already suffer from 'lowered mental ability' because of iodine disorders.[18]

At a national level, the estimated prevalence of 'endemic cretinism' plus 'milder mental/motor handicap' in Bhutan (22.31 per cent) and Nepal (12.84 per cent) must have significant effects on those tiny countries. Lower levels, such as in Sri Lanka (1.95 per cent ), Bangladesh (1.44 per cent) and Thailand (3.05 per cent), are not negligible.[19] Just from this single cause, the general prevalence of those recognized as suffering intellectual decline in Thailand has been doubled. The China National Committee on Care for Children estimates that 'IQ levels could be reduced by 10–15 points in eight million people' because of iodine deficiency.[20] In India, the UNICEF figure is 6.6 million children 'mildly retarded' and 2.2 million affected more seriously with cretinism.[21] These figures might be considered small in relation to the total populations in China and India, but those affected are in specific regions, not spread evenly throughout the country.

The estimated 120,000 Indian children born each year with iodine-related developmental disabilities represent a significant cost to the intellectual capital of particular regions.[22] In parts of Uttar Pradesh iodine deficiency affects 65 per cent of the population.[23] The Indian magazine *Frontline* reports that in Sikkim 16 per cent of the population is 'stunted, crippled "village idiots" some of whom cannot move more than an inch by themselves'.[24] In Nanpur, within a community of 4000 people, 90 per cent are reported to have goitre, known as 'galphor gaon'.[25] Is it surprising that such communities are also very poor?

> With every passing hour, there are at least ten children being born in India who will never attain their optimum mental or physical potential because of neonatal disorders caused by iodine deficiency.[26]

An alternative insight to that provided by simple prevalence rates comes from Hector Correa, who assessed the downward shift in average IQ caused by iodine deficiency in Ecuadorean villages.[27] He found that the average IQ stays at 100 until the percentage of goitrous people in a village exceeds 50 per cent. (Goitre in individuals suggests an accompanying mild intellectual dysfunction, and a high goitre prevalence in a population indicates an increase in more serious intellectual disability among some of that population.) Above this 50 per cent point, the average IQ starts to decrease as the percentage of goitrous people increases. The lowest average IQ Correa found was in the village of Guambalo, where it was 79. (Below 70 defines a clinical intellectual disability.) Rarely do statistics show such a clear 'break point' in relation to an environmental impact on the intellectual resources of a community, and it is probable that a similar effect could be identified in relation to other environmental causes.

Iodine deficiency is not the only form of 'hidden hunger' – it is simply the best documented. Zinc is also essential for optimum intellectual functioning. Between 65 and 75 per cent of people living in the Middle East and North Africa now get most of their calories from bread made from high-yield 'Green Revolution' wheat, which is low in essential zinc.[28] More than half the pregnant women in the world suffer iron-deficiency anaemia, which puts their babies at risk of impaired intellectual development.[29] About 56 per cent of pre-school children in India suffer levels of iron deficiency which are intellectually debilitating.[30]

Another concern of UNICEF is protein–energy malnutrition, which is a major cause of intellectual difficulties in developing countries. This affects over one-third of all children under 5 in the developing world.[31] In India, 43.8 per cent of children suffer moderate PEM; 8.7 per cent suffer an extreme level.[32] Land degradation resulting in poor crops is a significant cause of PEM.

Although the main concern has been the poorer nations, it is wrong to conclude that the 'hidden hunger' problem is not relevant elsewhere. In 1994, the Danish National Food Committee concluded that 75 per cent of Danish adults lack sufficient iodine, 50 per cent lack iron, 25 per cent calcium and 10 per cent folic acid. The cause is food fashion, in particular a move away from fish and green vegetables towards meat and dairy products.[33]

General malnutrition is the other perspective of *absence*-EMID, principally because it interferes with the brain fats which are necessary for proper brain development in young children. The Red Cross World Disaster Report concluded in 1996 that 'three-quarters of a billion people world-wide do not get enough food to live fully productive lives'. Again, although the poorer countries are the main concern, it would be wrong to assume that richer nations have no problems. A study from England and Wales found that some 47,500 low-birthweight babies were born in 1988. Ten per cent are expected to have a severe neuro-developmental handicap; a 'high proportion' of the remainder will have some form of deficit or disturbance.[34]

When one is assessing the effects of EMID it is crucial to ask not only 'how many?' and 'where?' but also 'who?' Often the impact is not evenly spread throughout a community. Poverty is without doubt related to increased exposure to environmental hazards. There is evidence that children from disadvantaged families suffer more than their wealthier peers from the effects of lead. They experience a greater fractional IQ loss and are more likely to end up in the 'borderline mentally handicapped' bracket.[35]

Similar inequity is apparent in relation to race. One major US study found that blood lead levels in black populations consistently exceeded those of white populations by 10 per cent in adults, 20 per cent in 6- to 17-year-olds and 40 per cent in under-fives. In part, the explanation stems from the condition of the home environment in the poorer areas inhabited by black populations, where lead in old paintwork and water pipes is common.[36] But poverty can provide a convenient explanation which can distract from the realization that much environmental victimization of minority groups is calculated, because of a belief that they will not resist. The US Commission for Racial Justice concludes that the racial make-up of a community is the 'most important' factor in the location of abandoned toxic waste sites in the USA.[37]

Figures concerning children in schools around Delhi who were goitrous owing to iodine deficiency provide a reminder that, even in the same geographical location, micronutrient status is greatly affected by economic status. In 1984 the *Indian Express* published a simple but telling comparison of prevalence in 'public' (i.e. fee-paying) schools and free government schools.[38] This Delhi report also contradicts the stereotyped view that iodine deficiency occurs only in remote rural areas.

|       | Public schools | Government schools |
|-------|----------------|--------------------|
| Boys  | 17%            | 42%                |
| Girls | 27%            | 60%                |

The discrepancy between boys and girls in both types of school is of equal interest to the wealth factor in this finding. Traditionally, in India, boys will usually be better fed than girls. The difference suggests that this is not just in relation to the quantity but also the quality of food – boys seemingly do better in terms of necessary micro-nutrients.

Gender does not often feature in the disaggregation of EMID. Professor Bryce-Smith of Reading University, the prominent UK anti-lead campaigner, points out that boys seem to suffer more severe brain damage from lead intake than girls.[39] This could relate to a greater time spent on the street, or to genetic vulnerability. Whatever the reason, this finding should cause educationalists to give some thought as to the possible link with statistics showing that boys constantly do worse than girls at school, and perhaps even with behaviour difference.

Prevalence statistics have many shortcomings. They are rarely based on straightforward head counts, but usually on generalizations from small population studies. They usually only relate to a single causatory factor. Epidemiologists may calculate that a third of the children in one region suffer intellectual decline from PEM, that 4 per cent suffer because of iodine deficiency and that 10 per cent have blood lead levels that threaten intelligence. But we would have no idea to what degree these figures relate to the same, or different, children.

There are not even statistics that view IDD and PEM together, yet this double impact is common in rural settings. Certain levels of chemical exposure may reduce IQ by only five or so points, but what of the additive effect of a number of different chemical exposures? What is happening in communities with a range of toxic threats *plus* poor nutrition where biological synergisms further the impact, as in the peri-urban 'shanty' settlements?

Currently it is only informal statements that provide any indication of the overall picture. A report concerning Katowice in Poland and Pibram in the Czech Republic talks of pollution 'doubling the number [of children] needing special education and halving those in the "exceptionally gifted" group'.[40] There are press reports that in four hundred villages near Unnao, India, 'More than 40 percent of the children . . . exhibit mild to advanced mental disability' owing to toxins in the water supply.[41]

Perhaps the most significant problem is that researchers may simply avoid assessments of EMID because they are too problematic, and because most medical statistics are based on counting the number of people treated. This can create a false impression that other, more readily identifiable environmental health impacts are more important. Hypothyroidism caused by deliberate releases of radioactive iodine from the nuclear facility at Hanford, Washington, has been linked to spontaneous abortions.[42] The

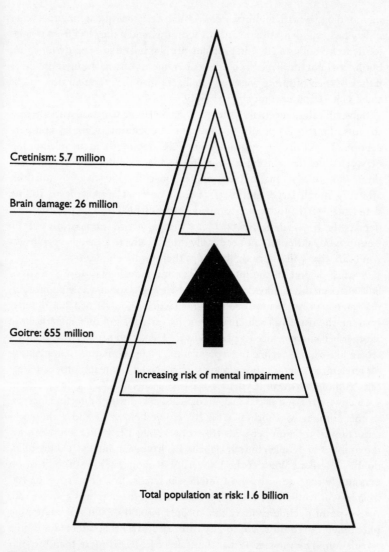

**Figure 2.1** Estimated impact of iodine deficiency worldwide. Even mild goitre (thyroid gland enlargement) is associated with some degree of mental impairment. *Source:* UNICEF, *State of the World's Children* (1995). Reproduced with permission.

methodology was straightforward. Women were sent questionnaires asking if they had experienced spontaneous abortions, and if they had been treated for hypothyroidism. Thyroid problems are also linked to brain dysfunction, but how could this have been assessed? A questionnaire asking individuals if they or their offspring were less intelligent than they thought they ought to be would not have much credibility.

Sub-clinical intellectual dysfunction eludes most statistical assessment – the loss of a few IQ points, or problems of cognition, memory and perception. The UNICEF pyramid (Figure 2.1) demonstrates the relationship between a defined clinical level of intellectual disability affecting a small proportion of a population, and milder sub-clinical levels of dysfunction affecting much larger numbers. This is not just applicable to iodine deficiency – it would relate to many forms of EMID. The pyramid also depicts the time-latent aspect. Many of the 'at risk' population will be parents who, although not necessarily directly affected, may have a health condition that will injure the brains of their future children.

A small decline in the intelligence of individuals may appear to have little effect on those individuals, but when viewed across a whole population, this can have a major impact on the intellectual resources of a community. Imagine the usual IQ bell curve centring on 100, and then superimpose another bell curve centred 5 points lower. The difference in overlap shows where sub-clinical decline hits a population. Françoise Barten, commenting on research in relation to lead exposure by Needleman and others, points out, 'Although a mean IQ deficit of 2 to 5 points may appear insignificant . . . a downward shift of this magnitude is associated with a threefold increase in the number of children with IQ scores below 80 and a threefold reduction in the number with IQ scores above 125.'[43] Put another way, the number of people clinically labelled as having an intellectual disability doubles. Bernard Weiss at the University of Rochester puts the situation graphically regarding the most intelligent sector. In a population of 100 million you would normally expect 2.3 million to have an IQ above 130. A five-point decline reduces this to only 990,000.[44] This demographic phenomenon would relate to any form of EMID that affected a whole population. The message is that the scale of EMID is more than the sum of the identifiable effects on individuals.

EMID is something that science demonstrates can happen, that local research shows does happen and that common sense suggests could be widespread in many communities. But the scale is virtually impossible to prove empirically, in the manner usually required to generate widespread concern. From existing statistical evidence, it would be difficult to argue that the environmental threat to the human intellect is global. But the effect on specific communities is without doubt acute. The question posed in

Chapter 1 – are the small-scale examples an indication of what is happening in larger populations? – must be answered less through head counts of those affected, and more from inferring an impact from what we know of the threat.

## Personal costs and consequences

There is nothing intrinsically undesirable about having an intellectual disability – provided the community in which you live has the willingness and capacity to make available the necessary support. People who are seen as having intellectual disabilities can hold down productive mainstream jobs, engage effectively in political processes, be good parents and safe drivers, and have many other qualities which permit them to make unique and valuable contributions to their communities. But, given the choice, we would all avoid any form of injury, whatever the outcome, and the proviso – necessary support – is a very significant one.

> I know I'm retarded. I know that can't be fixed. But if I could change myself . . . I wish I could be reborn. I don't want to be slow any more. I want to be fast. Sometimes I have dreams about it. I dream things like being able to tap dance or do ballet. But then I wake up. And I'm the same. I walk slow. I talk slow. My mind moves too slow. And sometimes that's harder than anybody understands. But I don't want to die. (Sandra Jensen, USA)[45]

Forms of so-called care in many countries leave no doubt as to the personal cost of intellectual disability. From Macau, near Hong Kong, Barry Grindrod reported on the 'forgotten cage-kids':

> *severely retarded young men and boys who spend their lives locked inside a pathetic, out-dated human zoo . . . Most of these spend a great part of their life in cages, the remainder usually pitiful vegetables lying in 40-year-old metal framed cots . . . a frightening noise comes from the corner of the large dimly lit room where a naked, young mute swings ape-like on the bars demanding bread as best he can.*[46]

In 1996, reports about Chinese orphanages from Human Rights Watch in Hong Kong claimed that children with severe intellectual disabilities were just left to die, without food or medical care. How many of these children were disabled because of environmental factors, such as China's unrivalled industrial pollution or iodine deficiency?

The relative wealth of particular countries does not necessarily mean more humane care. Sexual assaults and abuse, unlawful killings, muggings, theft and a spectrum of continuous low-level crime affect the lives of people with intellectual disabilities, even in relatively progressive countries such as Britain.[47] From Malaysia it was reported that at the Hope of Glory Hospital, 'one hundred retarded and physically disabled youths . . . are tied to beds which have no mattress, wallow in their own filth and are hosed down with water'.[48] While the victims who suffered intellectual disability because of mercury poisoning at Minamata Bay, Japan, were well provided for materially, their lives have been spent hidden away in institutions. They are a political embarrassment, and integrated care in the community has not been the Japanese approach to intellectual disability.

As communism came to an end in Eastern Europe, there were reports of similar circumstances, compounded by cold climates, from the Romanian, Russian and Albanian orphanages in which children were, and to a lesser degree still are, warehoused until an early death. The Cold War legacy is represented by a toxic industrial environment which destroys children's brains, and a concept of care that then destroys their dignity, health and eventually their lives. They are twice-victims of a war that was never fought.

An absence of religious belief was not to blame for inhumane attitudes in the former communist countries – the record of religion is very questionable. In 1981 a working party of the Anglican Church in Canada concluded:

> *Our senses and emotions lead us into the grave mistake of treating human-looking shapes as if they were human, although they lack the least vestige of human behaviour and intellect. In fact the only way to treat them humanely is not to treat them as human.*[49]

Within the Catholic Church it was not until 1983 that Communion became a right for those who could not express a belief in the Eucharist in words, which excluded many people with intellectual disabilities.

The dynamics of poverty, religion, national human rights abuses and war can distract from a more basic point. *Anyone* suffering intellectual decline in *any* country, however wealthy, is likely to suffer alienation. A US report about children born with disabilities because their mothers abuse drugs provides a recent example placed in historical context:

> *They have been called the 'children of the damned' and a 'biological underclass' . . . There is alarm at the term 'crack kid', which doctors fear unfairly stigmatizes the victims and will be as damaging as 'mongol' was to Down's syndrome children.*[50]

Myth can be as devastating as fact. When the Canadian press reported that Inuit people on Broughton Island had the highest levels of PCBs from pollution anywhere in the world, the outcome was that other Baffin

Islanders ostracized those they called the 'PCB people', and discouraged marriages to them.[51]

A UN Commission review, *Human Rights and the Environment*,[52] reminds us of another cost which brings the discussion full circle. Once disabled, an individual becomes more vulnerable to the other adverse outcomes of environmental change. The Commission proposes an 'unavoidable conclusion': 'the impact of the environment on disabled persons is felt at all stages, at several levels and in varying degrees – upstream as a cause of disability, and downstream by making the possibility of reintegration [into the community] more difficult'.

The personal cost of EMID therefore constitutes a double outcome: the injury itself and the social consequences of that form of injury. It is a cruel coincidence that the countries with the greatest environmental problems are usually also those with the least humane care systems for people with disabilities.

The broader personal cost is more apparent in the context of the ever-increasing demands for new and very specific intellectual skills, and in the light of 'jobless economic growth', which makes intellectual ability an ever-increasing determinate of survival in both formal and informal sectors. The world in which we now live expects forms of intellectual ability beyond the basic wisdom and common sense required to subsist through gathering, hunting, farming and animal husbandry. It is in this context that the 'sub-clinical' intellectual dysfunctions impact most, because they are unrecognized.

Illiteracy, for instance, is not intrinsically a threat to personal survival, until a significant number of the community becomes literate, which enhances their power over the remainder. That few individuals can now exist outside the cash economy makes a universal demand for numeracy, a very specialized intellectual skill that used not to underpin personal survival. Many indigenous African languages did not even have words for numbers. A few basic concepts such as 'one', 'both' and 'many' were adequate. Computer literacy is another new demand.

Even development strategies that prove effective with the very poorest communities require modern intellectual skills. The Grameen micro-banks in Bangladesh achieve exceptional success through providing small loans to two million people. There is only one criterion for getting a loan: the ability to understand how the bank works, which must be proved by passing an oral test. Not everyone passes, and of these many will be among the 1.44 per cent of the population who suffer intellectual decline because of iodine deficiency.

Within a century there has been a revolutionary change in what we now expect as the norm of intellectual functioning across the global population.

The result of these new intellectual demands is encapsulated by a simple but stark conclusion from the World Bank in 1991: that infants are more likely to survive if mothers have been formally educated. In previous eras this was not the case; in an equitable world it need not be the case. But in the real-world circumstances of today, survival increasingly equates with these new intellectual skills.

> Intelligence has become the new form of property. Focused intelligence, the ability to acquire and apply knowledge and know-how, is the new source of wealth. Singapore, which calls itself The Intelligent Island, recognizes that the traditional sources of wealth and competitive advantage – land, raw materials, money, and technology – can all be bought if needed, provided one has the intelligence and the know-how to apply them . . . The new source of wealth in our country is the intelligence quotient. Intelligence is, therefore, the new form of property. (Charles Handy, *The Age of Paradox*, Harvard Business School Press: Boston, 1994)

## Social costs and consequences

An outline of the social costs of EMID is the place for an important reminder. The 'costs' are *not* the costs of a disability: they are the costs of an environmentally mediated injury, which happens to cause a disability. The distinction is crucial. The result otherwise is to put new clothes on an old and dangerous philosophy: eugenics.

On the basis of human rights, the personal cost alone should be sufficient to inspire concern about intellectual decline. But history tells us that we are slow to address personal problems unless there is also a demonstrated social cost. The difficulty is that the standard methods for putting a price on social happenings are hard to apply. Robert F. Kennedy provided the argument in 1968:

> *The gross national product does not allow for the health of our children, the quality of their education or . . . the intelligence of our public debate . . . It measures neither our wisdom nor our learning . . . it measures everything, in short, except that which makes life worthwhile.*[53]

Put another way, mainstream economics fails to measure the human potential for positive survival.

But even in the crude economic terms required to influence governments, there are now a few useful arguments. In 1990 a US Congress report concluded: 'Neurotoxic chemicals constitute a major public health threat: the social and economic consequences of excessive exposure to them are very large.' More specifically, a 1985 study had estimated that the 'total health benefit of reducing the neurotoxic effects of lead on US children would amount to more than $500 million per annum', and this excludes the cost in relation to adults. It was also shown that reducing the maximum level of lead in tap water from 50 to 20 grams per litre would save $27.6 million in medical care and $81.2 million in special education.[54] New York has had to allocate a budget of $765 over the next ten years to meet the educational needs of children born with intellectual impairments because their mothers used crack during pregnancy.[55]

The National Research Council reports that the 'US Department of Health and Human Services has estimated that $23 billion was spent in 1980 for the care of people with diagnosed neurological diseases'. It then proposes, in broader terms, that 'it would not be surprising if the direct and indirect societal costs of subclinical neurologic losses or deficiencies – such as reduction in intelligence, diminution in achievement, and waste of opportunity – might equal or exceed those of neurotoxic effects that are clinically recognized'.[56] How such figures are generated is, of course, open to question. The point is less the degree to which such estimates are accurate, and more that statisticians are able to produce figures that *can* convince politicians of the need for action.

It is no surprise that this form of cash estimation is rarely made in relation to poor-nation *absence*-EMID. One exception is from the World Bank, which estimates that 'iron, vitamin A and iodine deficiencies are responsible for slicing as much as 5 per cent from the GDP of the developing world, enough to wipe out any economic growth in a low-income country'.[57] But there is little evidence that such assessments impact on national or global policy.

There is a clear incentive to avoid intellectual decline if the state picks up the bill for care – a 1995 estimate put the cost to the US state of a child born with Down's syndrome at $410,000 – but in most countries the state does not carry this burden. The awareness of social cost must therefore go well beyond the crude cash arguments required by rich-nation governments.

Cambodia demonstrates the difficulties posed to communities with a high prevalence of physical disabilities, owing in this case to land mines. But Cambodia also demonstrates that, with modest support, quite large numbers of people with physical disabilities are not an inherent burden on a community – often the reverse. The difficulties posed to communities by intellectual decline are different because it is not just day-to-day survival that is threatened. Social relationships that have long-term influences are likely to become confused – good decision-making, transferring knowledge, maintaining and developing cultural traditions. Those who do not suffer intellectual problems are likely eventually to leave such communities, compounding the problem.

## Families

Families face the biggest demands. Not least, they have to provide the direct care for disabled offspring, siblings and relatives. In poor countries the economic outcome is twofold: the cost of care and the loss of potential income. Families can show remarkable strengths in these circumstances, but this does not reduce the demands put upon them. In countries like India, it is not unknown for young people with intellectually disabled brothers or sisters to commit suicide because of the future burden that will, of tradition, be passed to them.

Diminished marriage opportunities are commonly recorded. Li and Wang report on a Chinese village, known as 'the village of the idiots', where iodine deficiency was so widespread that girls from other villages did not want to marry and live in the village.[58] Locals in Bhopal suspect that women injured by the Union Carbide poisoning will give birth to children with impairments, which diminishes marriage prospects. (And marriage brokers in India would put a very firm cash cost on this.) The situation can be exacerbated by careless press headlines such as one in the Indian *Sunday Observer*: 'Excess Fluoride Leaves in Its Wake a Village of Cretins.'[59] Attitudes towards the *hibakusha*, following the Hiroshima bomb, derived more from myth than scientific fact, but that did not alter the effect on families. Jay Lifton reported:

> [No one] can, with absolute scientific certainty, assure hibakusha that abnormalities will not eventually appear in their children, their grandchildren, or in still later generations . . . damage from radiation experienced by exposure in utero . . . resulted in a high incidence of microcephaly with and without mental retardation . . . Scientifically speaking, it has nothing to do with genetic problems. But ordinary people often fail to make the distinction: to them, children born with abnormally small heads and retarded minds seem still another example of the bomb's awesome capacity to inflict a physical curse upon its victims and their offspring.[60]

This situation is mirrored now by similar fears in the Chernobyl region.

The effect on marriageability also has implications beyond the family. Those suffering intellectual decline are likely to marry others of similar status. Consequently, any genetic damage is more likely to be transmitted to their children, because the same genetic mutation in both parents significantly increases the risk to the progeny. The response to difficulties in arranging marriages is often to opt for marriage to a relative.

Consanguinity (incest) is itself a major cause of intellectual disability, which may also be compounded by the genetic heritage of EMID.

## Education

In the past fifty years many of the newly independent countries have spent up to half their GDP on education. In regions where environmental factors diminish the educability of individuals, the expenditure is, in the terms of the Sufic tale, like pouring water into a leaking pot. What will be the impact of EMID on education and its relevance? Basil Hetzel reports that iodine deficiency in northern Indian villages creates 'a major block to human and social development'.[61] In affected areas there will be an increasing demand for a costly 'special needs' approach in schools, but this will compensate only to a limited degree. More specialist institutions will be needed, such as the Foundation for Children of the Copper Basin in Legnica, Poland, where an intensive, and expensive, detoxification programme has been set up to remove heavy metals from the bodies of schoolchildren (see Chapter 8). A US Environmental Protection Agency estimation in 1985 projected a 1990 cost of $309 million for compensatory education and $107 million for medical care (1983 dollars), if leaded petrol continued to be used.[62] And these costs related to only a single toxin in a rich country which already had relatively high standards of protection.

There is a further educational Catch-22. Much of our intellectual ability develops through interaction with our family and immediate peers. Sadly, but realistically, those who suffer intellectual decline in the poorer countries are likely to gravitate into social and familial proximity. If the intellectual resources of a social environment are low, such communities consequently enter a degenerative spiral.

Education ministries should now be in the front line of environmental activism, but ministerial divides intervene. Do education ministers, in countries with high levels of iodine deficiency, ever use the prevalence statistics when determining education policy priorities? It seems improbable, because such statistics are the domain of health ministers. Why does the UK Department for Education and Employment not question the fact that the British standard for lead in drinking water is less strict than that set by the World Health Organization, by a factor of five? In many cities, a significant aspect of excessive car use is taking children to school – adding to the lead and other pollution which reduces school achievement. Which ministry would take, and act on, a comprehensive view of this situation? There are obvious disincentives, not least that this year's Minister for Education might be next year's Minister of the Environment.

## Public order

The exploitation of individuals with intellectual difficulties, which leads to anti-social behaviour, is a necessary concern but one that is hard to argue without conclusions that blame the victim. If there is a danger of this discussion appearing as new-age eugenics, this is where it is most likely to happen. But the eugenics movement sometimes founded its inhuman arguments on human truths, and these should not become unavailable to other forms of discussion just because they are tainted.

While there is absolutely no evidence that people with intellectual disabilities are inherently criminal, individuals of low intelligence, just above the level of a clinical disability, can be susceptible to anti-social influence. In the words of a British policeman, 'They're just bright enough to follow instructions, and just stupid enough to do as they're told.' One British study discovered that the average IQ of suspects in police cells was 82.[63] Another found that a quarter of those in UK prisons have learning difficulties – twice the national average.[64] The Cambridge Study in Delinquent Development concludes, 'children with low intelligence are more likely to offend because they tend to fail at school and hence cannot achieve their goals legally'.[65] Hyperactivity, impulsivity (attention-deficit syndrome) and difficulty manipulating abstract concepts are all linked to an increased likelihood of delinquency,[66] and these problems have all been linked, in part, to exposure to environmental chemicals. But there is really little need for extensive academic research to make clear the connection between petty crime and low intelligence. A few hours sitting in any local courtroom is sufficiently persuasive.

On a more serious level, Adrian Raine argues that birth complications causing mild brain damage, which may go unnoticed in early life, *combined* with parental rejection, predispose boys to violent behaviour in adulthood. Boys with drowsy brain wave patterns 'were significantly more likely to end up with criminal records at the age of 24'.[67] Raine concludes that avoiding birth complications 'could help reduce violent crime by more than 20 percent in the next generation'. And exploitation can go beyond crime. From South Africa there were reports of the use of mentally handicapped men as 'special combat units' of the fundamentalist, racist sect Israel Vision.

## National development

Intellectual resources are a missing factor in development theory, except for the education perspective, which is largely based on dubious measurables such as exam achievement, enrolment and attendance. We rarely think beyond visible indicators of development – wealth, housing, health, clean water, food, clothing, participatory governance – to take account of the invisible: the intellectual potential within communities which provides the *fundamental* ability for individuals to achieve positive development.

Communities affected by EMID are almost certainly likely to suffer economic problems. Back in 1975, Frank Gilfillan produced a very intriguing argument that lead poisoning contributed to the fall of the Roman Empire.[68] Whether right or wrong in relation to Rome, the reasoning Gilfillan uses could well be applied to contemporary settings. Why, for example, when Bihar has 80 per cent of India's mineral wealth, is it now one of the poorest states in the country? In 1500 BC it was the principal state in northern India. Is it a coincidence that the region also suffers significantly from iodine depletion, and more recently from unregulated factory pollution, such as mercury from Bihar Caustic and Chemicals Ltd which has caused environmental contamination 81 per cent above WHO guidelines?

UNICEF talks of iodine deficiency 'locking entire communities into a vicious cycle of ineducability and poverty'.[69] Researchers from the Programme against Micronutrient Malnutrition provide an impression of the situation in the Philippines: 'The result is poor productivity; a nation not up to par economically; a substandard quality of life for its citizens; and a community which cannot compete globally.'[70] On a local level, Li and Wang report of a Chinese community where 'the economic development of the village was retarded' and there was no truck driver or teacher.[71] A more formal assessment of the effects of iodine deficiency in Ecuador found a strong relationship between intellectual decline and personal income. In a community where the average IQ had sunk from 100 to 79, the average personal income halved.[72]

The scenario does not just apply to poorer nations. Kathryn Mahaffey, of the US National Institute of Environmental Health Sciences, reminds us of consequences which all governments should heed in relation to just one threat, lead:

> *In coming decades, maximizing the intellectual and educational capacity of our population will be critical to our success in dealing with many social and economic challenges. The importance of safeguarding the intellectual and educational development of our children against preventable disease is difficult to overestimate. Childhood exposure to lead is preventable. The data [now available] . . . emphasize the intellectual cost of not preventing it.*[73]

The time-latent nature of EMID puts its impact well beyond the scope of traditional economic prediction.

The UN warns of another cost to development within communities with low intellectual resources. 'Although they may seem much less obvious than any physical disability, learning disorders are a particular source of danger because they may affect an entire population and even impair its capacity to resist exploitation.'[74] The outcomes of iodine deficiency, described by Hetzel, include 'a high degree of apathy' (even affecting domestic animals) and 'effects on initiative and decision-making'.[75] In the villages of Unnau, India, not only is a high level of disability evident, but there are few village headmen and villagers cannot remember when they last had a village meeting. Education and health services have long since disappeared, and, unsurprisingly, there seems little incentive among the villagers to redress this exploitation. Development theories lauding the value of 'participation', 'empowerment', 'rights-based approaches' and 'mobilization' require considerable qualification in the light of EMID. In some settings benign paternalism may well be the most workable short-term option to prevent the demise of communities.

Affected communities will probably not be able to organize themselves to resist environmental exploitation such as the adjacent siting of toxic factories and dumps. There is ample evidence that it is poorer, often minority group, communities that suffer intellectual decline and other environmental health problems, because of this form of exploitation. The degenerative spiral is easy to envisage.

The ultimate outcome is that 'false norms' arise in communities with a high prevalence of intellectual disability: the circumstance becomes accepted.[76] Regions of nineteenth-century Switzerland, where IDD-related cretinism was very prevalent, provide a historical example. Those who suffered were considered to represent a blessing from God, and families were thought to be on bad terms with heaven if no family members were affected. A contemporary parallel is not dissimilar. Researchers from the Programme against Micronutrient Malnutrition report from the Philippines: 'IDD is so commonplace that many feel it is a normal part of life'.[77]

But to put outcomes in such neat compartments can be misleading. The real concern is unexpected compound consequences. As described earlier, a single environmental cause, which has a hardly detectable impact of five IQ points on individuals, has a marked effect on a population and can strike in a surprising way at a number of aspects of community cohesion. The tripling of the numbers of those with an IQ of around 80 relates directly to the problem of criminality mentioned above. And the threefold reduction around IQ 125 depletes a human resource cadre at a level of greatest scarcity for most countries: the intelligent, technically competent workforce. A minor sub-clinical effect from a single pollutant can constitute a compound economic blow to the community that suffers. In poorer countries, the link between intellectual potential, literacy and birth rates can have a similar compounding effect in relation to many of the standard variables of development theory, yet EMID never features as a factor.

The standard assumptions of interrelatedness in development theory have omitted intellectual decline as a variable, yet links are not complicated. For example:

● Poverty is both cause and effect of high birth rates. *Intellectual decline leads to economic decline and an inability to manage the environment sustainably, which increases poverty, which fuels high birth rates.*
● Female illiteracy is linked to high birth rates. *Illiteracy (and an absence of non-literate family planning skills) will be greater in communities suffering intellectual decline, precipitating high birth rates and poverty.*
● High birth rates mean that populations grow beyond the capacity of the environment to feed them, and poor nutrition results. *Poor nutrition causes intellectual decline, which, through illiteracy, may precipitate high birth rates and poverty.*
● Polluting industries and toxic dumps are often sited near poor communities. Pollution, and poor nutrition owing to poisoned farmland, cause intellectual decline, which reduces the community's ability to resist further exploitation. *Exploitation compounds the spiral of poverty, poor nutrition, high birth rates, illiteracy and intellectual decline.*

The most important aspect of cost in relation to a community is also probably the most difficult to accept. Putting aside personal and family perspectives, injury is usually a greater cost to a community than death, and intellectual impairment is probably a greater burden than physical injury. Consider why so many weapons of war are intended to injure, not kill. Land mines are the obvious example, and some are designed to jump into the air and explode at head level specifically to cause brain and sensory damage.

The apparent decline in male fertility provides a broader example. If new environmental chemicals *kill* human sperm and reduce fertility, in global terms this might solve a major problem – overpopulation. The 'cost' is at an interpersonal level. But if these new chemicals also *injure* sperm, causing widespread intellectual decline and other impairments, we have a major cost consequence from global to local levels.

What we fear most immediately is not extinction, but the insidious erosion of the human species. We worry about an invisible loss of human potential. We worry about the power of hormone-disrupting chemicals to undermine and alter the characteristics that make us uniquely human – our behaviour, intelligence, and capacity for social organization. The scientific evidence about the impact of hormone disruptors on brain development and behaviour may shed new light on some of the troubling trends we are witnessing.[78]

## Notes

1. National Research Council, *Environmental Neurotoxicology* (National Academy Press: Washington, DC, 1992), p. 17.

2. D.J. Weatherall, *The New Genetics and Clinical Practice* (Oxford University Press: Oxford, 1991), p. 30.

3. M. Al-Ansari, 'Etiology of mild mental retardation among Bahraini children: a community-based case control study', *Mental Retardation* (1993), **31**(3), 140–3.

4. IDRC, *Environmental Management Development in Ukraine: Dnipro River Basin* (International Development Research Centre: Ottawa, 1994).

5. M.D. Chivian et al., *Critical Condition: Human Health and the Environment* (MIT Press: Cambridge, MA, 1993).

6. Sierra Club, *e-mail Bulletin*, 30 May 1996.

7. Alexander Dorozynski, 'Paris finds high lead concentrations in its poorer children', *British Medical Journal* (1993), **307**, 523.

8. Alison Motluk, 'Lead blights the future of Africa's children', *New Scientist* (1996), **2022**, 6.

9. Geoffrey Lean, 'The greedy cities', *Independent on Sunday*, 14 April 1996, p. 17.

10. Murray Feshbach and Alfred Friendly, *Ecocide in the USSR: Health and Nature under Siege* (Aurum Press: London, 1992), pp. 9, 10, 11, 66, 67, 92, 184.

11. Françoise Barten, *Environmental Lead Exposure of Children in Managua, Nicaragua: An Urban Health Problem* (CIP-Gegevens Koninklijke Bibliotheek: The Hague, 1992), p. 61.

12. World Bank, *Environmental Action Programme for Central and Eastern Europe* (Ministerial Conference: Lucerne, 1993), Annex 1, p. 1.

13. W.J. Rogan et al., 'Congenital poisoning by polychlorinated biphenyls and their contaminants in Taiwan', *Science* (1988), **241**, 334–6.

14. Theo Colborn, Dianne Dumanoski and John Peterson Myers, *Our Stolen Future* (Little, Brown & Co.: London, 1996), p. 235.

15. G. Greig, 'Crack kids give America a new lesson in suffering', *Sunday Times* (8 March 1992), p. 21.

16. Jane Seymour, 'Hungry for a new revolution', *New Scientist* (1996), **2023**, 37.

17. UNICEF, *Annual Report* (UNICEF: New York, 1994), p. 51.

18. UNICEF, *The State of the World's Children 1995* (UNICEF: New York, 1995), pp.18, 15.

19. Basil Hetzel, *The Story of Iodine Deficiency* (Oxford University Press: Oxford, 1989).

20. Richard Tomlinson, 'Eight million Chinese with reduced IQ because of iodine shortage', *British Medical Journal* (1995), **310**, 146.

21. Jon Bliot Rodhe, '6m Indian kids have damaged brain', *Newstime*, Hyderabad, 3 October 1993.

22. ICCIDD, 'Iodine deficiency causes 30,000 still births', *Indian Express*, 19 March 1994.

23. GEAG, *Iodine Deficiency in Trans Saryu Plains: Health Problems* (UNICEF: Gorakpur, 1993).

24. Frontline, 'Sikim's sorrow', *Frontline*, India, 14 August 1992, pp. 98–104.

25. Probe India, 'The goitre gaon', *Probe India* (1992), June, pp. 28–32.

26. 'Frightening information', *Times of India*, 19 January 1994.

27. Hector Correa, 'A cost–benefit study of iodine supplementation programme for the prevention of endemic goitre and cretinism', in J.B. Stanbury and B.S. Hetzel, *Endemic Goitre and Cretinism: Iodine Nutrition in Health and Disease* (John Wiley & Sons: New York, 1980), p. 577.

28. Seymour, *op. cit.* (n. 16), 36

29. UNICEF, *op. cit.* (n. 18), p. 19.

30. UNICEF, *The Right to Be a Child* (UNICEF: Delhi, 1994), p. 12.

31. UNICEF, *op. cit.* (n. 18), p. 17.

32. UNICEF, *op. cit.* (n. 30), p. 12.

33. Margaret Dolley, 'Denmark to tackle high goitre rate by adding iodine to salt', *British Medical Journal*, 30 July 1994, p. 309.

34. M.A. Crawford *et al.*, 'Essential fatty acids in early development', in U. Bracco and R.J. Deckelbaum (eds), *Polyunsaturated Fatty Acids in Human Nutrition* (Raven Press: New York, 1992).

35. Kathryn R. Mahaffey, 'Exposure to lead in childhood', *New England Journal of Medicine*, **327** (18), 1308–9.

36. R. Lansdown and W. Yule, *Lead Toxicity*, Johns Hopkins University Press: Baltimore, 1986), p. 114.

37. Richard Hofrichter, *Toxic Struggles: The Theory and Practice of Environmental Justice* (New Society Publishers: Philadelphia, 1993), p. 27.

38. *Indian Express*, 31 January 1984, p. 5.

39. Liz Hodgkinson, 'Overactive ingredients in boys and girls', *The Times*, 8 August 1991.

40. Diane Seligsohn, 'Insidious poisoner at home', *The European*, 4–10 February 1994, p. 16.

41. Rajiv Saxena, 'Excess fluoride leaves in its wake a village of cretins', *Sunday Observer*, India, 15–21 December 1991, p. 3.

42. C.M. Grossman and R.H. Nussbaum, 'Hypothyroidism and spontaneous abortions among Hanford, Washington, downwinders', *Environmental Health* (1996), May/June, 175–6.

43. Françoise Barten, *op. cit.* (n. 11), p. 15.

44. Colborn *et al.*, *op. cit.* (n. 14), p. 236

45. Kevin Toolis, 'A heart for Jo', *Guardian Weekend*, 10 August 1996, p. 23.

46. Christopher Williams, *The Right to Be Known: A Global View of Human Rights and Mental Handicap* (Norah Fry Research Centre, University of Bristol: Bristol, 1993).

47. Christopher Williams, *Invisible Victims: Crime and Abuse against People with Learning Disabilities* (Jessica Kingsley Publishers: London, 1995).

48. Williams, *op. cit* (n. 46), p. 34.

49. *Ibid.*, p. 5.

50. Greig, *op. cit.* (n. 15), p. 21.

51. Colborn *et al.*, *op. cit.* (n. 14), p. 108

52. UN, *Human Rights and the Environment* (UN Commission on Human Rights: New York, 1994), para. 150.

53. Ismail Serageldin and Andrew Steer (eds), *Making Development Sustainable: From Concepts to Action* (The World Bank: Washington, DC, 1994), p.17.

54. Office of Technology Assessment, US Congress, *Neurotoxicity: Identifying and Controlling Poisons of the Nervous System*, OTA-BA-436 (US Government Printing Office: Washington, DC, 1990) pp. iii, 20, 230–1.

55. Greig, *op. cit.* (n. 15), p. 21.

56. National Research Council, *op. cit.* (n. 1), p. 18.

57. Seymour, *op. cit.* (n. 16), 36.

58. J.Q. Li and X. Wang, 'Jixian: a success story in IDD control', *IDD Newsletter* (1987), **3** (1), 4–5.

59. Saxena, *op. cit.* (n. 41), p. 3.

60. Robert Jay Lifton, *Death in Life: The Survivors of Hiroshima* (Weidenfeld & Nicolson: London, 1967), p. 106.

61. Hetzel, *op. cit.* (n. 19), p. 92.

62. J. Schwartz *et al.*, *Costs & Benefits of Reducing Lead in Gasoline. Final Regulatory Impact Analysis*, EPA 230-05-006 (EPA: Washington, DC, 1985).

63. Gisli Gudjonsson, Isabel Clare, Susan Rutter and John Pearse, *Persons at Risk during Interviews in Police Custody: The Identification of Vulnerabilities* (HMSO: London, 1993).

64. Angela Devlin, *Criminal Classes* (Waterside Press: Winchester, 1994).

65. David P. Farrington, 'The origins of the crime: the Cambridge study in delinquent development', *Research Bulletin (Home Office)* (1989), **27**, 29–32.

66. David Farrington, *Understanding and Preventing Youth Crime* (Joseph Rowntree Foundation: York, 1996).

67. Steve Connor, 'Crimes of violence: birth of a solution', *Independent*, 8 March 1994, p. 19.

68. Frank Gilfillan, 'Lead poisoning and the fall of Rome', *Journal of Occupational Medicine* (1975), **7**, 53–60.

69. UNICEF, *The State of the World's Children* (UNICEF: New York, 1990), p. 36.

70. PAMM, 'Misconception of IDD prevalence obstacle to strong legislation', *PAMM News* (1995), January, 2.

71. J.Q. Li and X. Wang, *op. cit.* (n. 58), 4–5.

72. Correa, *op. cit.* (n. 27), p. 577.

73. Mahaffey, *op. cit.* (n. 35), 1308–9.

74. UN, *Document E/CN.4 Sub 2/1991/31* (UN: New York, 1991), p. 37.

75. Hetzel, *op. cit.* (n. 19), p. 92.

76. Christopher Williams, 'An environmental victimology', *Social Problems* (1996), **23**(4).

77. PAMM, *op. cit.* (n. 70), 2.

78. Colborn *et al.*, *op. cit.* (n. 14), p. 234.

# The Bodily Environment

# CHAPTER 3

# The Mobile Environment of the Brain: Medical Science

'The body is the mobile environment of the brain.' Buckminster Fuller reminds us that we represent a mini-ecosystem within which the brain exists in mutual cooperation with the whole.[1] The message from environmentalists is how little we know about the ecosystem and the consequences of human-made change. In contrast, we are now complacent about the power of medical science to understand and cure the dysfunctions of the human body. But when the two are viewed together – the brain is put at the centre of a bodily environment within our global environment – it becomes clear that we know too little about these relationships to assess with confidence the environmental threat to human intelligence.

What is 'intellectual decline', how is it assessed and what are the limitations of assessment? What are the threats to intelligence viewed from a medical perspective within the *absence–presence–synergism* paradigm? How do the 'protective sciences' function and are they serving us well?

## What is intellectual decline?

On a single day in 1973, 8 million US citizens were suddenly not 'mentally retarded'. This was not divine intervention – the definition for 'borderline mentally retarded' had been moved down one standard deviation and as a result the official prevalence rate was reduced from 3 to 1 per cent. Intellectual impairment is more a social construct than a medical condition. Below an arbitrary line individuals take on the label of 'clinical' intellectual disability, with sub-divisions such as profound, severe, moderate and mild. Above that line there is a range of so-called 'sub-clinical' forms of intellectual dysfunction. Some of these are milder versions of clinical conditions; some are unrelated and may be seen as an additional aspect of a clinical condition. The need to construct categories is not solely Western – the Zulu words *isilima* and *isiphoxo* describe respectively severe and mild intellectual disabilities.[2]

There is a broad agreement about what constitutes 'clinical' intellectual disability, and that this derives from a prenatal condition – often labelled 'birth defect' or 'birth injury' – or an event in early childhood. The World Health Organization provides the standard definition: 'intellectual functioning that is significantly below average' *combined with* 'marked impairment in the ability of the individual to adapt to the daily demands of the social environment'.[3] The disability also arises because of the inability of society to adapt to that individual. Put more practically, a term like 'severe mental handicap' probably describes people who may never learn to eat, read and write, clean their teeth or go to the toilet without help. Acquired brain injury – caused, for example, by accidents, occupational-related toxins and, arguably, drug and alcohol abuse – can leave individuals with impairments that are very similar to those stemming from infancy.

The 'sub-clinical' dysfunctions do not necessarily have their roots in early life, and impact on intellectual functioning in direct and indirect ways. Rachel Carson recorded in *Silent Spring* a description of non-permanent, sub-clinical effects from two British scientists who had deliberately dosed themselves with DDT:

> *The tiredness, heaviness, and aching of limbs were very real things, and the mental state was also most distressing . . . [there was] extreme irritability . . . great distaste for work of any sort . . . a feeling of mental incompetence in tackling the simplest mental task.*[4]

It is not hard to imagine the effect on a whole workforce suffering symptoms of this nature, even in a very mild form. In the wealthy southern suburbs of Mexico City pollution-related morning lethargy is now widely recognized, as people find it increasingly hard to get out of bed and be active at the start of the day.

Another important aspect is physical disability and illness, which, although not clinically impairing the brain, can impact on the intellectual development of children in certain circumstances. Childhood arthritis can affect the regions of the brain dealing with spatial cognition, because these regions are not stimulated owing to reduced limb movement. Blindness, which may be caused by vitamin A deficiency, is a more obvious example. The link between physical impairments and intellectual development is less evident in the wealthy countries, where special education and clinical remediation are usually widely available, but it is significant in poorer countries.

Neurotoxins that do not directly impair the intellect can impact indirectly. Schoolchildren who become 'distracted', 'disorganized' or 'frustrated', or who 'cannot follow simple instructions', all because of lead poisoning, seem unlikely to optimize their intellectual potential. Disrupted motor skills together with memory deficits might have a greater impact in China, where the ability to learn and write over two thousand characters at a young age forms the basis for literacy. Remembering that intelligence is largely our *potential* to learn and adapt, these indirect threats are a crucial part of the overall picture.

Neuro-degenerative diseases associated with old age may be linked with environmental exposures, but this form of decline is rarely perceived as an aspect of a nation's intellectual resources, simply as a potential cost to the welfare state. Dr Peter Evans, working at the University of Cambridge, concludes that 'cognitive deficits appearing in later life may not be directly caused by senility or the ageing process itself, but may be the result of developmental deficits or toxic damage which has occurred several decades earlier'.[5] A link is being made between Alzheimer's disease and aluminium exposure.[6] Researchers at Aberdeen University add another dimension. From studies of people who grew up in poor mining families decades ago, it seems that poor nutrition also precipitates Alzheimer's. People who suffer both nutritional deficiencies and exposure to environmental toxins may be at even greater risk.

As nerve and brain cells do not regenerate, any loss is additive. (There are compensating mechanisms, so loss does not correlate directly with intellectual ability.) The demise of a few cells owing to environmental factors may appear 'sub-clinical' in mid-life; so too might a natural loss in later life. But when these are added together, the outcome may, according to the US National Research Council, be a significant decline in intellectual functioning.[7]

But it is misleading to envision brain impairment as simply loss of organic matter. Damage is better perceived as a disruption of the brain's processing abilities. Quite large chunks of the brain can be removed with surprisingly little impact on intelligence, but a minute toxic insult in the right place at the right time can create a major impairment. The jazz trumpeter may perform perfectly on an aged instrument that is battered, scratched and dented, yet a speck of dirt in a valve can render it instantly unplayable.

## Assessing intellectual decline

Western psychology provides numerous techniques for measuring intelligence and related brain functions, loosely termed 'developmental tests'. Briefly, tests for infants note developmental stages such as eye contact and holding the head up. Tests for young children consist of simple tasks such as putting square shapes into square holes and round shapes into round holes. Tests for older children assess reasoning through quasi-literate skills and eventually formal literacy and numeracy. New forms of test are being developed in relation to dementia in old age.[8]

Intelligence quotient (IQ) tests provide a score for an individual in relation to the average of a population (IQ 100), with respect to age. The importance is to recognize the limitations of these tests. The margin of error in IQ testing is around 15 points – IQ 70 could mean anything from 55 to 85. In general, intelligence testing is very questionable in relation to individuals, but is useful when assessing effects across populations. The arguments about what exactly IQ tests measure are infinite. But we can say with some certainty that whatever is being measured, people who have more of it usually enjoy less problematic lives than those with less.

A common criticism is the cultural inappropriateness of many tests. Picture cards still used to test British children show dogs and pigs. The latter would be abhorrent to a Jewish child, and any depiction of living creatures would be improper to a Muslim. In the 1970s it was found that half the Mexican-American children in San Francisco who were put in classes for 'mentally retarded' children had average or above average scores when culturally appropriate tests were used.[9] Cultural variation can be overcome. In New Guinea, a test of psychomotor skills that required children to tighten a nut was incomprehensible, but a test based on threading beads worked very well.[10]

There is a further complication, which is not addressed in the medical textbooks. How do you measure intellectual decline, resulting from an environmental cause, in someone who has a pre-existing intellectual disability? While the problem may appear marginal to medical theory, it is very real in the polluted world in which many people must now live. Take one example. Children with an intellectual disability often have a behaviour trait known as *pica* – they eat non-food substances such as soil. In a shanty town in the proximity of a smelter, where soil may be heavily contaminated with heavy metals, a child with a naturally occurring intellectual disability may suffer further decline by eating soil.[11] This is unlikely to be detected as a condition caused by the smelter, yet it is as much an injury to a child with a pre-existing intellectual disability as it is to one with no disability. A child with one arm who loses another because of a land mine is seen clearly as a victim; a child with Down's syndrome who suffers further intellectual decline because of a lead smelter is not.

## The threats to the intellect
### *Presence*-EMID
Environmental threats to the brain, caused by the *presence* of toxic agents, are usefully categorized by the pioneer UK scientist and anti-lead campaigner Derek Bryce-Smith:[12]

1 *Genotoxins*, which cause genetic changes in sperm or ova that lead to disturbances of the brain of the unborn child following conception, or chromosome abnormalities causing conditions such as Down's syndrome, e.g. some pesticides, ethylene dibromide and lead (both are petrol additives) or ionizing radiation. Heritable effects are either somatic (parent–child) or germ-line (transmittable to other future generations).

2 *Teratogens*, which cause injury directly to the brain of the foetus and are usually transferred via the mother's body or stem from a pre-conception exposure of the mother or father, e.g. alcohol, smoking, cocaine, lead, methylmercury, carbon monoxide, some pesticides, dioxin, solvents such as toluene, probably benzene, ionizing radiation.

3 *Neurotoxins*, which create disorders after birth, including (possibly) degenerative disease, e.g. lead, methylmercury, aluminium, cadmium, arsenic, carbon monoxide, some pesticides, solvents such as toluene, ionizing radiation.

But the clarity of this typology should not lead to an impression that scientific knowledge is complete. The UN SCOPE committee concludes: 'Screening tests for potential neurotoxins must be viewed as less than satisfactory.'[13] Current typologies show us where and how to look, but do not reveal the extent of what might be seen.

Lead appears in all three groups and is a principle cause of *presence*-EMID. Our awareness of its danger is not new. Pliny (AD 23 to 79) noted the neurotoxic impact of lead, which was used in wine-making at that time. It is worth understanding the nature of lead poisoning more fully, because it provides an indication of the nature of many of the other threats. Like many neurotoxins, but unlike other metals such as copper or zinc, lead serves no physiological purpose for humans. Any exposure, however small, is therefore an unnatural interference within the bodily environment. The important characteristics are:

- infants and children absorb lead more readily than adults;

- lead appears in blood and urine within hours, and then accumulates in the liver, bone, fatty tissue and brain;

- lead transfers from mother to foetus very readily across the placenta;

- the outcome appears dose-related – the greater the body burden of lead the more severe the intellectual decline;

- the ingestion of regular small amounts in the long term can be as significant as acute poisoning in the short term;

- outcomes range from death and severe visible disabilities (encephalopathy and hydrocephalus), to serious 'clinical' intellectual disabilities, to 'sub-clinical' IQ deficits and behavioural problems.

Ionizing radiation rarely appears within the ambit of neurotoxicology because radiation is not strictly a toxin. More correctly, it creates a toxic effect in the body. Significant data appeared in 1990, derived from the Japanese survivors of the Hiroshima and Nagasaki A-bomb.[14] There was no evidence of severe retardation in those exposed at less than the 7 weeks' gestation stage, but this is probably because the damage to very vulnerable cells was so great that pregnancies terminated. The relative risk for those exposed in the 8- to 15-week period was four times greater than that for exposure at 16 to 25 weeks after conception. A dose of 1 sievert results in severe mental retardation (IQ less than 70 in this interpretation) in about 40 per cent of those exposed. A similar pattern relates to IQ scores, with a dose relationship of about 30 IQ points per sievert. Measures of school performance showed a slight variation from this pattern: those in both the 8 to 15 and the 16 to 25 week groups showed 'a highly significant decrease in school achievement'. Those exposed before 7 weeks and after 26 showed no evidence of effect. There is a very clear relationship between increased dose and increased percentages of children born with severe mental retardation or small head size.

> The frequency of severe mental retardation in Japanese A-bomb survivors exposed at 8–15 weeks of gestational age has been found to increase more steeply with dose than was expected . . . [Data] imply that there may be little, if any, threshold for the effect when the brain is in its most sensitive stage of development. Pending further information, the risk of this type of injury to the developing embryo must not be overlooked in assessing the health implications of low-level exposure for women of childbearing age.[15]

Intellectual decline caused by the exposure of the infant brain *after* birth has been established following research on children with brain tumours or leukaemia who have been treated therapeutically with ionizing radiation. One study concludes: 'significant reductions were found in overall intelligence score for the majority of children, younger patients being most affected'. Other studies show that children who were treated with radiation had memory defects, lower examination scores, fewer school grades completed and clinical mental retardation.[16]

The body's natural defence mechanisms, which prevent neurotoxins attacking the brain, are a crucial but often forgotten aspect of *presence*-EMID. The defences provided by the liver and kidney are the most obvious, and many toxic insults are immediately stored in body fats and bone and released slowly only in minute amounts to be dealt with in a controlled way. Environmental toxins can damage these defences, opening the door to direct impacts on the brain.

In *Silent Spring*, Rachel Carson points out that a chemical such as methoxychlor, which can affect the brain after long exposure, is stored in the body at 100 times its normal rate if the liver has already been damaged by another insecticide.[17] Neurotoxins such as mercury, cadmium and lead can cause kidney damage, which then permits these same substances to reach the brain more easily. Research from the University of Birmingham in the UK proposes that Parkinson's and motor neurone disease might be precipitated because of a failure of the body to break down toxic chemicals such as pesticides into harmless water-soluble forms that can be excreted. The failure may arise because of damage to the bodily defences by other environmental toxins.[18] Although these two conditions do not impair the intellect, the mechanism could be similar for forms of dementia such as Alzheimer's disease.

The blood–brain barrier – a continuous lining of special cells – restricts the entry of potentially dangerous molecules from the bloodstream to the brain. Similarly, the nose–brain barrier defends against airborne threats; the veins in the nose connect directly with those in the brain. The blood–brain barrier can be breached by lipophilic substances (body fats) and therefore toxins can reach the brain if they are lipid-soluble or structurally similar to other substances that are normally taken up by the brain. Sniffing gasoline (intentionally or otherwise) permits lead to reach the brain more quickly than ingestion because this organic form of lead is fat-soluble and penetrates the blood–brain barrier more easily than inorganic forms. Irradiation of the central nervous system may increase the permeability of the blood–brain barrier, and cause liver or kidney damage.

For the unborn child, the placenta provides a protective barrier, but this defence is limited. Lead, for example, is readily transferred across the placenta from the twelfth week of pregnancy. The blood–brain barrier is not completely formed at birth, and less so in premature infants, so there is a particular vulnerability at this time.

Damage to the nasal defences provides a unique aspect, because the nose also functions as an early warning system for direct toxins. The initially unpleasant smell of organic solvents, for example, tells us to avoid high levels of inhalation. But extended exposure to a solvent such as toluene not only interferes with brain functioning, but also reduces our ability to smell the solvent,[19] and therefore our instinct to avoid the threat is rendered inoperative.

The list of environmental agents causing *presence*-EMID is therefore considerably greater if we include chemicals that damage our bodily defences against the direct neurotoxins.

## *Absence*-EMID and psycho-social deprivation

General nutrition is clearly linked to intellectual development. In poor rural areas the absence of adequate food is increasingly caused by environmental degradation. Malnourished mothers are more likely to produce babies of low birth weight, which causes intellectual problems, and women who eat less than 1700 calories each day will probably have children with intellectual disabilities.[20] Malnutrition during the tenth to eighteenth weeks of pregnancy leads to the birth of a child who has fewer brain cells. Brain size is not directly linked to intelligence in individuals but there is a broad correlation across populations, and people with larger brains seem less likely to suffer dementia in later life.

Malnutrition in infancy leads to a 15 to 20 per cent deficit in brain cells, and poor development of the interconnections between nerve cells, axons and synapses, which can be compounded by lack of social stimulation. The initial belief that the connection between malnutrition and intellectual development is a simple matter of clinical cause-and-effect has now been challenged. It is realized that the influences of poverty, illness and social factors – all within an interrelated cause–effect–cause spiral – are extremely complex.[21] For example, children who are small through undernourishment may be treated as infants within a family, which affects their intellectual development even if there is no obvious brain impairment.

Until recently, obvious malnutrition – the images of famine and starvation – has overshadowed the effects of less obvious micro-nutrient deficiencies. There may be enough to eat – but does the soil in which this food is grown, and the type of food, create the balance of micro-nutrients required for proper human development? Much of this 'hidden hunger' stems from subtle forms of environmental degradation – excessive flooding caused by deforestation can wash vital micro-nutrients from the soil, for example. Other problems stem from the Green Revolution. New crop varieties have caused iron, zinc, vitamin A and other micro-nutrient deficiencies.[22] Iron-deficiency anaemia reduces work capacity in adults, retards foetal growth if pregnant women suffer and weakens cognitive ability in infants. Many of the hidden hunger problems do not directly damage the brain, but those affected simply do not have the energy to learn or use their brains in an optimum manner.

> [There] is another malnutrition which is not visible, either to parents or health workers or to a world-wide public . . . It is the malnutrition of the child who is sitting in the shade, dull-eyed, without even the energy to ward off the flies, of the child who rarely joins in the games of others, of the child whose eyes are glazed over behind a school desk and who does not understand what he or she is being taught. Protein–energy malnutrition means disruption in the miraculous process by which neurons migrate to the right location in the brain and begin to form the billions of subtle synapses that make lifelong learning possible.[23]

The global campaign against iodine deficiency has not yet proposed that redressing ecological degradation should be a long-term strategy to address the problem, focusing on more immediate mitigation such as the iodizing of salt. This view stems, in part, from the history of iodine deficiency, which was originally largely associated with remote rural populations living in mountainous European regions where iodine had leached naturally from the soil. It is now starting to be acknowledged by medical writers that much iodine deficiency in poorer nations stems from human-caused environmental degradation, fuelled by population increase and forced migration to remote areas.[24]

> Human beings need only a teaspoonful of iodine in their diet over a whole lifetime. But insufficient iodine can result in irreversible damage to brain and body. In high terrain and wherever rainfall or floods wash iodine from the soil, children grow up stunted, mentally retarded, apathetic, and incapable of normal movement, speech or hearing. Severe iodine deficiency at birth places children at risk of cretinism. Even mild deficiency shows up later in life as poor performance at school and poor productivity in adulthood.[25]

Nutritional deficiencies are not entirely a poor-nation problem. Michael Crawford and his team at the Institute of Brain Chemistry and Human Nutrition in London point out that, in countries where there has been such a keen interest about health problems caused by unessential fats (mainly heart disease), it is paradoxical that so little attention has been given to problems for brain development caused by deficiencies of *essential* fats. The brain is held together by structural lipids, and deficiency of fatty acids during early development causes permanent impairment.[26] Maternal nutrition and smoking before conception are important factors. Micro-nutrient deficiency can also arise in rich nations. The same team found significant problems in East London caused by a lack of dietary magnesium.[27]

There is another important form of *absence*-EMID. To a psychologist, talk of 'the environment' in relation to the development of human intelligence would not initially create a vision of the chemical–biological hazards that are the main concern of *Terminus Brain*. The first thought would be of problems caused by a child's psycho-social environment – the absence of supportive parenting, restricted interaction with peers, an unstimulating home life, a lack of education, no toys – all of which are clearly related to restricted cognitive and other intellectual development. One South African study re-emphasizes the importance of a strong mother-bond for infants. Irrespective of poverty, securely bonded infants do better developmentally. The precocity of many African infants has been linked to child-rearing customs which include specific stimulation and handling of infants.[28]

A poor psycho-social environment can create a form of intellectual disability that is virtually indistinguishable from that arising from other organic causes. In one widely documented example, two Czech twins were cruelly treated and spent most of their childhood locked in a cellar. Although when found they were, in appearance, significantly mentally handicapped, remediation was so effective that eventually their intellectual progress was virtually normal.

Oppressive child labour can have an impact. In a sporting goods factory in Sialkot, Pakistan, children aged five upwards are made to work 80 hours a week, with one half-hour meal break each day, *in total silence*. The manager claims, 'If the children speak, they are not giving their complete attention to the product and liable to make errors.'[29] There is no need for a battery of psychological tests to work out the probable results of communication deprivation on intellectual development.

In some circumstances, the absence of appropriate social and physical environments might alter the brain organically. Animal research has shown that putting rats in an enriched environment, with wheels and mazes, can lead to larger cerebral cortices, bigger neurons, more active neurotransmitters and larger blood supplies to the brain, within a month. The increase is greatest with younger rats, but older ones show some change, and females are affected more than males. It follows that a restricted psycho-social environment might have the reverse effect, and perhaps that females would suffer most. There are still no firm conclusions about the degree to which the psycho-social environment brings about physical change in the brain, as distinct from inhibiting the optimum potential of the brain machinery as it exists. But these studies raise interesting questions about unstimulating lifestyles. What, for example, is the effect of long-term unemployment, particularly in the rich nations, where the result is usually a dreary home-bound life not so dissimilar from that of a mouse in a cage?

There has long been a debate about whether the psycho-social or chemical environment is the greater determinant of individual intelligence. But in the real-world context it is less important to assess which perspective is more correct than to realize that both play a part. In the homes of the world's poor it is not difficult to see how, for example, a sub-clinical dulling of a child's intellect by lead from a kerosene stove, which might be compounded by nutritional deficiencies, can easily become a significant disability because of an unstimulating psycho-social environment. The child then enters a degenerative spiral, unable to resist the social dynamics or self-stimulate, excluded from formal education and the chance of free school meals and health care, because intellectual ability is the entry ticket to school, and so spending even more time in the polluted and unstimulating home.

There could be a further chemical–social synergism. If, as the authors of *Our Stolen Future*[30] argue, new synthetic chemicals in the environment are interfering with the ability of animals to rear their young, could they have the same effect on humans? If so, the same chemical soup may represent a double blow to intellectual development: as a direct neurotoxin, but also through disrupting parenting and therefore the psycho-social environment of home.

But perhaps the most significant characteristic of the psycho-social aspect is how it demonstrates the rich world–poor world research divide. Psycho-social research in the rich nations has examined in minute detail causal relationships that might have a fractional effect on children's development, yet in contrast we know virtually nothing of the widespread environmental brain poisoning of the poor. Researchers in the rich countries examine whether listening to music can enhance children's intelligence. We even know that it is better to play children Mozart than Mick Jagger on our stereos. Yet we know little of the effect of environmental mercury on thousands of native children in the Amazon basin: a threat that arises from mining the gold that pays for the stereo systems and CDs that might notch up the intelligence of the wealthy a few micro-points.

## Adverse synergism

Adverse synergisms are a major part of the EMID aetiology, but are ignored because clinical assessment is problematic. *Absence*-precipitated synergism seems common. In non-scientific terms, it is easy to envisage an organism that needs to take in certain elements for its survival, which, when it cannot get those elements, instead takes in other similar elements, which may be harmful, in an attempt to rectify the deficiency. The human body seems to do much the same when placed in the unbalanced environments that we have now created. Iron, vitamin D and calcium deficiencies seem to precipitate lead absorption. Calcium deficiency increases absorption of radioactive strontium, which behaves like calcium. Zinc deficiency is a direct cause of intellectual decline, but a zinc-deficient body will also try to compensate by absorbing increased levels of other, perhaps toxic, metals.

There seem also to be a few *presence*-precipitated synergisms. Excessive levels of zinc or cadmium can exacerbate copper deficiency, which is a relatively rare condition in a balanced environment.[31] Causes are sometimes not so obscure. Eating only brown rice binds iron in the body in a way that causes deficiencies of that mineral. High alcohol consumption fools the body into believing that it has taken in normal nutrients, so reducing the absorption of those vital minerals and vitamins in their normal form.

Additive effect – presence plus presence – is also part of adverse synergism. If an individual is exposed to methylmercury and lead, the impact on the brain is likely to be greater than from a single substance. But the effects are not simply additive – they are also sometimes interactive. Small amounts of an organophosphorus insecticide, fenitrothion, can react with DDT to cause liver damage, leading to brain impairment which mimics Reye's syndrome.[32] In the 1970s, car painters in Finland suffered memory loss because of exposure to a range of 'safe' solvents, which when combined affected the brain. Synergisms can also be additive *and* interactive. From experiments on mice it seems that the presence of cadmium in the body compounds the effects of lead, but it also seems to interfere with the way in which the body regulates zinc, thus perhaps creating an internal deficiency even if the environmental supply is adequate.[33]

It would be convenient if the bodily environment always functioned in the neat compartments suggested above. But of course this is not always so. The body's natural defences also play their part in adverse synergism.

In the Democratic Republic of Congo (formerly Zaire), cassava is a staple food. If it is carelessly prepared or eaten excessively, the result is cyanide poisoning. This is dealt with by a defence, the liver, which produces high levels of thiocyanate in the blood. This thiocyanate causes an excessive loss of iodine through the kidneys, and then possibly intellectual decline caused by iodine deficiency. If the same individuals happen to live in regions where there is an absence of iodine in the environment, there is also a compounding effect leading to a greater chance of hypothyroidism and intellectual decline.[34]

Intergenerational synergism can combine all aspects. A woman who has been exposed to lead in younger life may have absorbed lead into her bones – a mechanism representing a natural defence against the lead reaching her brain. But if she becomes pregnant, and her unborn child suffers a calcium deficiency, it will take calcium from the mother's bones – together with the lead – across the placenta defence. In this simple example there is an adverse synergism between *absence* and *presence*, which happens because of one of the body's natural defence mechanisms and then defeats a reproductive defence.

Biological synergism becomes more significant when viewed in the social context of poorer countries. The *absence* of necessary environmental agents is usually seen as a rural problem; the *presence* of environmental toxins, urban. But in the ever-growing informal settlements – the 'shanty towns' – around the cities of the poorer countries both problems come together.

The converse is also the case. Many dirty industries which require a small labour force, such as nuclear power stations, are deliberately sited in rural areas within poorer countries. Local people, who probably already suffer (rural) nutritional deficiencies, are exposed to high levels of industrial (urban) pollutants, such as lead from shielding and protective clothing discarded around the nuclear power stations. In addition, other pollution can degrade farmland, creating further micro-nutrient problems.

Social environments create and compound the adverse synergisms within the bodily environment. Probably the most pressing job for environmental medicine in the future is to escape from single-substance science and understand what happens to the human brain in synergistic settings. As yet there are few scientists exploring the crucial field of 'toxico-dietics'.[35] The reason is simple: interdisciplinary science is an unwise career move.

The medical paradigm of EMID is multifaceted but not complicated. An understanding of the general picture does not require a knowledge of obscure science (Figure 3.1). It derives more from remembering dynamics that are currently peripheral because of a research bias towards easy, clear-cut clinical impacts. To a scientist, research in an informal settlement is messy because of the compounding synergism, and best left to someone else. To a policy-maker, the informal settlements should be the conceptual starting-point of strategies to ensure the security of a nation's intellectual resources.

## Establishing cause and effect: the protective sciences

Toxicology, human biology, epidemiology and reproductive medicine are the main 'protective sciences' standing between the human brain and the threats posed by environmental agents. Experimental science – how does it happen in humans? – contributes to the observational science of epidemiology – did it happen in a population? – to establish cause and effect. The result should be a robust form of risk assessment leading to the

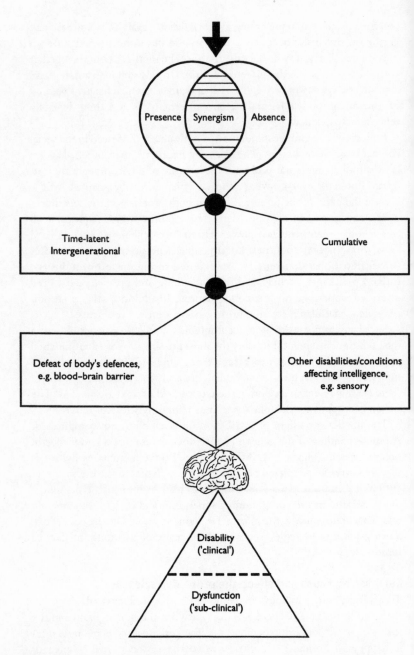

**Figure 3.1**   The medical dynamics of EMID.

minimization of hazards. But current environmental methods, derived largely in relation to cancer, are starting to be seen as very inadequate when applied to the brain.

## Toxicology and *presence*-EMID

Common household salt appears on standard lists of workplace reproductive hazards. Presumably this is because splitting salt into caustic soda and chlorine gas causes it to become dangerously toxic, but the apparent absurdity emphasizes that toxicology has to go well beyond listing potentially hazardous substances if it is to relate to the real world. The techniques of toxicology fall into four spheres.

First are *human studies*, which are rare. Ideal research would involve the deliberate exposure of humans to known doses of potential neurotoxins, which is obviously not acceptable. (But there are examples, such as work by US scientists in relation to radiation at the start of the Cold War.) Most human data stem from opportunistic research following industrial accidents, but levels of exposure are often unclear. This means that human data are scarce and often very dated. Current risk assessment in relation to mercury still relies heavily on studies following the Chisso poisoning at Minamata Bay, Japan, in the 1950s. The presence of toxins can be detected in the short term in blood and urine, in the long term in teeth, bone or fingernails, and dated in hair samples.

Second, *animal studies* form the basis of most evaluations. These usually entail giving very high doses of a substance to animals and inferring low-dose effects in humans, which is obviously problematic. Results vary widely between animals. A minute amount of dioxin can kill a guinea pig, yet a hamster will survive a dose 5000 times greater.[36] In addition, the toxins used in animal experiments are often not in the same form as the toxins in the environment. Research regarding lead does not use lead in the form in which it is used in petrol, for example. *In vitro ('test tube') animal studies* provide a third aspect, which can determine the site of action or mechanism of action, indicating the possible effects in humans.

Unfortunately, humans and animals do not always function in the same way. Thalidomide, which caused severe physical and some mental impairments in human babies, showed no effect when tested on animals. Animal studies might work reasonably well for outcomes such as cancer, which are readily diagnosable and involve the observation of effects on organs, such as the liver, which are broadly comparable between rodents and humans. But comparisons are much more problematic in the determination of intellectual decline. The brains of mice and men are very different. Although simple psychological experiments are possible, you cannot ask a mouse to take an IQ test.

Fourth are studies on *toxicokinetics and toxicodynamics*, which are very limited. It is rarely possible to tell if a substance will harm the human brain from looking at its chemical structure alone. The hitherto commonly used 'structure–activity relationship' (SAR) method, which has worked well concerning other hazards, is now deemed 'a poor basis for predicting neurotoxic potential'.[37] Almost any environmental agent, if present in the right amount, at the right place, at the right time in human development, could cause some form of intellectual impairment. Understanding the mechanisms of exposure, and finding the biological markers – the 'footprints' left by toxics *en route* – which can help to identify the mechanisms, is probably more important than understanding the chemical nature of specific environmental agents.

Studies of *genetic predisposition* – ecogenetics – are providing new perspectives.[38] Some individuals may be less able to render toxins harmless, through normal body functions, and therefore more susceptible to potentially neurotoxic effects. Non-genetic predisposition poses another aspect. According to the US National Research Council, 'few compounds have been assessed for selective toxicity to vulnerable groups within the population, such as the very young and very old'.[39] Laboratory work can never replicate the real-life situation of human populations.

> Extrapolations from animal data involve making inferences from a healthy, properly fed, genetically homogeneous animal population to a human population which includes groups which vary in age, health, and nutritional status, and is generally heterogeneous. Similarly, human data, when available, are often derived from a working population of healthy adults, usually male.[40]

Whether it is owing to inadequate scientific methods or inadequate implementation of existing methods, the result is that we know very little about potential neurotoxins. There are 3.5 million known chemicals. Between 60,000 and 70,000 are acknowledged to be in commercial use, and usage is increasing by around 5000 each year. It has become a cliché to point out how few of the chemicals in daily use have been tested for their effects on humans, but when the end-point is the human brain, the situation seems exponentially worse.

The lack of scientific understanding of how the brain will survive in the context of current human-caused environmental change provides one of the strongest arguments for the precautionary principle.

[Except] for pharmaceuticals, less than 10% of the chemicals in commerce have been tested at all for neurotoxicity, and only a handful have been evaluated thoroughly . . . 5% of all industrial chemicals, excluding pesticides, are likely to be neurotoxic . . . Furthermore, resources are not readily available to undertake across-the-board testing of all chemical substances already in commerce . . . There is a particular lack of data on chronic and long-latency neurotoxic effects.[41]

## Human biology and *absence*-EMID

The establishment of *absence*-EMID through the understandings of human biology makes use of a similar mix of animal and human studies. Detecting *absence* is sometimes more difficult than detecting *presence*. While hair and blood samples are valuable to establish the intake of toxins, they are not, for instance, good indicators of zinc deficiency. Testing methods can also be subjective. One way of determining if individuals suffer from zinc deficiency is to give them a weak solution of zinc in water; if they report that it tastes 'just like water', zinc deficiency is suspected.[42] This is not to say that such techniques are inappropriate, just a reminder that some aspects of scientific method rely greatly on human perception.

It is misleading to envisage biologists as simply trying to detect the effects of a total absence of micro-nutrients. More accurately, they are usually seeking to assess the effects of an *imbalance*. For example, too little vitamin A causes blindness, too much in pregnant mothers leads to birth impairments and the right amount seems to prevent some cancers. Both vitamins A and B$_6$ are vital to the body as trace elements, but become neurotoxic in large amounts. Hence treatments for deficiency, if not well regulated, can be iatrogenic − cures that cause ills.

## Epidemiology

Epidemiology links what is known or suspected as a result of toxicological or biological studies with effects in populations. The standard weaknesses of environmental epidemiology are that the exposed population is usually small, the outcomes are rare events and exposure is usually poorly defined. Add to this that there may be a number of environmental causes and contributory factors culminating in single outcomes in individuals, or multifaceted outcomes from a single agent.

In relation to EMID, there are other specific difficulties. Most significant is that the outcome is largely a social construct, part of a continuum and therefore open to wide interpretation, and is significantly influenced by non-chemical factors such as parenting or education. While outcomes such as anophthalmia (children born with no eyes) are finite, intellectual decline is not, and the problem of detecting EMID in someone who has a pre-existing intellectual disability is virtually impossible to overcome. For these reasons most epidemiological studies of EMID attend to what is easiest – the readily recognizable conditions such as Down's syndrome – omitting the probably much more widespread but less tangible outcomes.

There are also difficulties in relating degree of exposure to an environmental agent to severity of outcome: 'dose response', which is considered a strong indicator of cause and effect. It is particularly hard to assess dose response when the outcome is severe, because it is difficult to rank severity in those with an IQ of less than 60. Very high *in utero* toxic exposures may cause brain-related death of the foetus rather than brain impairments, which would be suffered at lower doses. The level of intellectual decline in unborn children following high levels of radiation exposure may appear small because the foetuses naturally abort. Human factors also intervene. Following the nuclear industry disaster at Chernobyl, many mothers opted for abortions, thus statistically reducing the birth impairments attributable to radiation.

Time-latency creates significant problems. Many intellectual disabilities caused by reproductive problems will not become apparent until years later. Severe mental retardation caused by the nuclear industry disaster at Chernobyl would not be detectable until infants were aged two[43]. Because a female's eggs are formed in the ovaries when she is still a foetus, it is a pregnant woman's *grandchildren* who may be the victims of her exposure to environmental agents. It is not adequate simply to base statistics on prevalence at a certain point, because many of those born with disabilities will not exist in older populations, as they will die in infancy owing to their inherent weakness, or even suffer infanticide.[44]

It is not surprising that the epidemiological method provides ready arguments for those wishing to refute links. It is all too easy to conclude, 'Needs more research'. Canada's Atomic Energy Control Board provides an example:

> With respect to the elevated rates of Down [sic] Syndrome, the report concluded that any possible relationship with tritium releases was weak and contradictory. Further research was recommended to verify mother's residence at the time of birth of the Down Syndrome cases, and to examine other possible contributing factors such as medical X-ray exposures and occupations of both parents.[45]

The efficacy of epidemiology is even less in poorer countries, where scarce resources, expertise and cultural variation compound the standard difficulties. Yet this is also where the environmental threats are usually greatest.

## Reproductive medicine

Reproductive medicine develops the lessons of experimental and observational science in relation to childbirth. The key concepts are:

- *mutagenic* effects, or changes in genetic material of or transmitted via the sperm or ova;

- *teratogenic* effects, or other birth impairments or developmental abnormalities caused by a direct impact on the embryo or foetus;

- *deficiencies* of micro-nutrients, such as iodine or folic acid, which are common causes of birth impairments.

Many of the general difficulties of toxicology and biology apply to reproductive perspectives. For example, by 1981, only 3 per cent of the chemicals known to be teratogenic in animals were known to have the same effect on humans.[46] The importance of reproductive health is the particular vulnerability of the unborn child. Concerning mercury, for example, blood levels in the foetus are about 28 per cent higher than in its mother, and concentration in the brain is four times higher.

Toxins in breast milk are an increasing concern. It has been known for many years that acute exposures to substances such as methylmercury can lead to contamination of milk, and even higher levels of the toxin in the breast-fed baby than in the mother. More recently there has been a debate about accumulation of general environmental toxins such as PCBs.[47] The conundrum this poses is whether or not the hazard from contamination of breast milk is greater than intellectual decline from not feeding naturally (about eight IQ points). The dilemma is compounded further by the toxins in cows' milk used to make the substitutes.

The main interest of reproductive medicine has traditionally been women, but this is misguided. Reproductive hazards are also transmitted through men. For instance, it has long been known that male agricultural workers may suffer levels of exposure to pesticides that affect their sperm, leading to birth problems.[48]

Another missing component from reproductive medicine is child labour, especially in relation to pre-puberty. Occupational reproductive health has not considered, for instance, the effects of pesticides on the ova of the 10-year-old girl working in the Colombian flower-growing industry. Safety levels have been set assuming only adult male exposure.

In *Our Stolen Future*, Theo Colborn argues that the most significant new area of concern is the probable threat posed by the new synthetic hormone-disrupting chemicals. Effects have long been noted in wild animals and laboratory experiments, but these hazards do not fit the standard paradigms of reproductive medicine because they are not genetic and do not attack DNA. As a consequence they have been largely ignored (see Appendix).

A baby's intelligence depends as much on the levels of thyroid hormone reaching the brain during critical periods of development as on inheriting smart genes . . . synthetic chemicals can obstruct the hormone messages during prenatal development and permanently alter the outcome . . .

Extensive research on the developing brain and nervous system has found that thyroid hormones help orchestrate the elaborate step-by-step process that is required for normal brain development . . . These hormones stimulate the proliferation of nerve cells and later guide the orderly migration of nerve cells to appropriate areas of the brain . . . When thyroid levels are too high or too low, this development process will go awry and permanent damage will result, which can range from mental retardation to more subtle behavioural disorders and learning disabilities.

Hormone systems do not behave according to the classical dose-response model that informs our thinking about biological responses to perturbations . . . where the biological response to a foreign substance increases as the dose becomes greater . . . The response does not necessarily continue to increase as the dose increases . . . high doses may, in fact, produce less of an effect than lower doses.

. . . There is an urgent need to look for 'impaired function' as well as for disorders that fit the classic notions of disease. For example, having a poor short-term memory or difficulty in paying attention because of exposure to PCBs is very different from having a brain tumour. The former . . . can have serious consequences over a lifetime and for a society. They erode human potential and undermine the quality of human life.[49]

Perhaps the most crucial question for reproductive medicine to answer in the future is: can we infer from the death of sperm and ova that there will be a concomitant level of brain injury because of lesser damage to sperm and ovum that is insufficient to kill but sufficient to damage? Marijuana use is one possible example. Death of sperm or ova is easy to measure, and often seen to relate to environmental factors. For example, the ongoing reduction in sperm counts may well be connected to the presence of environmental chemicals, such as phthalates, which mimic oestrogen. If the link between cell death and cell damage is established, it may provide the aetiology for much hitherto unexplained intellectual and other impairment at birth.

## Not proven

This outline of the limitations of the protective sciences does not derive from campaign groups or the media. Sources are mostly conservative: mainstream findings from international, governmental and quasi-governmental research organizations exemplified from the established scientific journals. Yet the obvious conclusion appears alarmist: current scientific methods attempting to establish causation in relation to EMID are uniquely problematic and may well remain so, and consequently we have very little conclusive evidence.

This seems to lead in one of two directions. We ignore the minimal evidence that exists on the basis that we require a large quantity of firm data; otherwise the verdict is 'not guilty'. Or we take very seriously such scarce evidence as exists, principally because it is scarce, and adopt a 'guilty until proven innocent' view of environmental threats – a precautionary principle. The reluctance to do this stems in part from the possibility of retrospective damages claims if common chemicals are suddenly put on the suspect list. There is, however, another verdict between guilty and not guilty, which the Scottish courts occasionally apply: 'not proven'. On one occasion this was explained by a canny judge to a joyful defendant as 'Not guilty – but don't do it again.'

It seems that protective science cannot yet keep up with the problems caused by the over-extensive application of progressive science. The next chapter therefore poses the obvious question: might science of the future present a different picture, especially in relation to 'risk assessment'?

## Notes

1. R. Buckminster Fuller, *Utopia or Oblivion* (Bantam Books: New York, 1969), p. 367.

2. Leonard Bloom, 'Some psychological concepts of urban Africans', *Ethnology* (1964), **3**, 66–95.

3. WHO, *Mental Retardation: Meeting the Challenge* (World Health Organization: Geneva, 1985), p. 8.

4. Rachel Carson, *Silent Spring* (Pelican: Harmondsworth, 1982), p. 172.

5. P.H. Evans, 'Nutrient and toxin interactions in neurodegenerative disease', *Proceedings of the Nutrition Society* (1994), **53**, 431–42.

6. National Research Council, *Environmental Neurotoxicology* (National Academy Press: Washington, DC, 1992), p. 15. P.H. Evans, E. Yano, E. Peterhans and J. Klinowski, 'Aluminium and trace elementoxidative interactions in the etiopathogenesis of Alzheimer's disease', in A. Favier and P. Faure, *Trace Elements and Free Radicals in Oxidative Diseases* (AOCS Press: London, 1994).

7. National Research Council, *Environmental Neurotoxicology* (National Academy Press: Washington, DC, 1992), p. 31.

8. J.P. Das and R.K. Mishra, 'Assessment of cognitive decline associated with aging: a comparison of individuals with Down Syndrome and other etiologies', *Research in Developmental Disabilities* (1995), **16**(1), 11–25.

9. James Herndon, *How to Survive in Your Native Land* (Bantam Books: New York, 1985), p. 96.

10. Basil S. Hetzel, *The Story of Iodine Deficiency* (Oxford University Press: Oxford, 1989), p. 66.

11. Françoise Barton, *Environmental Lead Exposure of Children in Managua, Nicaragua: An Urban Health Problem* (CIP-Gegevens Koninklijke Bibliotheek: The Hague, 1993), p. 83.

12. D. Bryce-Smith, 'Heavy metals and brain function', in A. Wynn-Jones (ed.), *Nutritional, Chemical and Para-medical Influences on Mental Retardation* (MENCAP: Taunton, 1985).

13. H.J. Fallon, 'Methods of clinical surveillance: effects on the liver and other organs', in V.B. Vouk *et al*. (eds), *Methods for Assessing the Effects of Mixtures of Chemicals* (John Wiley & Sons: New York, 1987), p. 330.

14. National Research Council, *Health Effects of Exposure to Low Levels of Ionizing Radiation* (BEIR V) (National Academic Press: Washington, DC, 1990), pp. 7, 83, 355–61.

15. National Research Council *op. cit*. (n. 14).

16. UNSCEAR, *Sources and Effects of Ionizing Radiation* (United Nations: New York, 1993), p. 827.

17. Carson, *op. cit*. (n. 4), p. 175.

18. Rosemary Waring, Letter, *The Lancet*, 12 August 1989, pp. 356–7.

19. Donna Mergler and Brigitte Beauvais, 'Olfactory threshold shift following controlled 7-hour exposure to toluene and/or xylene', *NeuroToxicology* (1992), **13**, 211–16.

20. John Elkington, *The Poisoned Womb* (Pelican: Harmondsworth, 1985), p. 22.

21. J.L. Brown and E. Pollitt, 'Malnutrition, poverty and intellectual development', *Scientific American* (1996), **274**(2), 26–31.

22. Jane Seymour, 'Hungry for a new revolution', *New Scientist* (1996), **2023**, 32–7.

23. UNICEF, *The State of the World's Children* (UNICEF: New York, 1995), pp. 16–17.

24. A.J. McMichael, *Planetary Overload: Global Environmental Change and the Health of the Human Species* (Cambridge University Press: Cambridge, 1993), p. 210.

25. UNICEF, *The State of the World's Children* (UNICEF: New York, 1993), p. 36.

26. M.A. Crawford *et al*., 'Essential fatty acids in early development', in U. Bracco and R.J. Deckelbaum (eds), *Polyunsaturated Fatty Acids in Human Nutrition* (Raven Press: New York, 1992).

27. W. Doyle, *et al*., 'Maternal magnesium intake and pregnancy outcome', *Magnesium Research* (1989), **2**(3), 205–10.

28. S. Harkness and C.M. Super, 'The developmental niche: a theoretical framework for analysing the household production of health', *Social Science and Medicine* (1990), **6**, 23–32.

29. Jonathan Silvers, 'When they were very young', *Independent on Sunday*, 28 April 1996, pp. 6–7.

30. Theo Colborn, Dianne Dumanoski and John Peterson Myers, *Our Stolen Future* (Little, Brown & Co.: London, 1996).

31. Elizabeth Green, 'The value of diet and mineral supplements for mentally retarded people', in A. Wynn-Jones (ed.), *Nutritional, Chemical and Para-medical Influences on Mental Retardation* (MENCAP: Taunton, 1995).

32. Christopher Robbins, *Poisoned Harvest* (Victor Gollancz: London, 1991), p. 42.

33. Elkington, *op. cit*. (n. 20), pp. 114, 208.

34. Hetzel, *op. cit*. (n. 10), p. 45.

35. P.H. Evans, 'Nutrient and toxin interactions in neurodegenerative disease', *Proceedings of the Nutrition Society* (1994), **53**, 431–42.

36. Joseph V. Rodericks, *Calculated Risks: The Toxicity and Human Health Risks of Chemicals in Our Environment* (Cambridge University Press: Cambridge, 1992), p. 54.

37. NRC, *Environmental Neurotoxicology*, (National Academy Press: Washington, DC, 1992), p. 124.

38. Philippe Grandjean, *Ecogenetics: Genetic Predisposition to the Toxic Effects of Chemicals* (WHO/Chapman & Hall: London, 1992).

39. NRC, *op. cit.* (n. 37), p. 17.

40. V.B. Vouk and P.J. Sheenhan, *Methods for Assessing the Effects of Mixtures of Chemicals* (John Wiley & Sons: New York, 1987), p. 736.

41. NRC, *op. cit.* (n. 37), pp. 2, 3, 17.

42. Bryce-Smith, *op. cit.* (n. 12).

43. David R. Marples, *The Social Impact of the Chernobyl Disaster* (St Martin's Press: New York, 1988), p. 53.

44. W.L. Langer, 'Infanticide: a historical survey', *History and Childhood* (1986), **1**, 353.

45. AECB, *Tritium Releases from the Pickering Nuclear Generating Station and Birth Defects and Infant Mortality in Nearby Communities 1971–1988* (Atomic Energy Control Board: Ottawa, 1991), p. 4.

46. R.B. Kurzel and C.L. Cetrulo, 'The effect of environmental pollutants on human reproduction, including birth defects', *Environmental Science and Technology* (1981), **15**, 626.

47. Deborah Baldwin, 'The all-natural diet isn't', *Environmental Action* (1992), **9**(15), 2–6.

48. R. Balarajan and M. McDowall, 'Congenital malformations and agricultural workers', *The Lancet*, 14 May 1983, p. 1112.

49. Colborn *et al.*, *op. cit.* (n. 30), pp. 206–8, 187.

# CHAPTER 4

# Protective Science: The Long Term

As recently as 1976, scientists maintained that the link between brain impairment and lead was 'not proven'.[1] Now the US Centers for Disease Control in Atlanta consider lead 'the most common and psychically devastating environmental disease of young children'.[2] It is a truism to say that science is constantly changing, but it is a truism that begs the question: why does science sometimes not seem to acknowledge this?

Scientific fact is rarely presented in a time framework, yet this is crucial when discussion concerns fast-changing environmental threats and fast-changing protective sciences. What are the trends in the foreseeable future? Where is science going and how might this change our perception of EMID, especially in relation to risk assessment?

Looking beyond the foreseeable future and analysing the situation more theoretically over an *infinite* time scale presents two paradoxes. One stems from a question of intergenerational justice: might the protective sciences, particularly the way risk is assessed, perpetuate a form of intergenerational eugenics? The other derives from a possibility that scientific progress, as both cause and cure of the problem, seems set to destroy the evidence needed to establish that there is a problem.

### Future trends
#### Assessing effect
The area in which the future will be least like the present is probably the identification of brain impairment. Sensitive scanning equipment is now able to detect forms of dysfunction, whether from disease or toxic chemicals, that could not be seen a decade ago. Functional magnetic resonance imaging can now provide a high-definition moving picture of brain activity in real time, and is non-invasive and much safer than X-rays. One recent result is a new understanding from the National Institutes of Health in Bethesda, Maryland, that dyslexia arises from differences in brain function that exist before birth. This increases the possibility that environmental agents could, in some circumstances, be a causal factor.

Genetic techniques being developed at the Oxford Institute of Molecular Medicine will permit the identification of idiopathic intellectual disability, through viewing sub-microscopic exchanges of genetic material (DNA) at the tips of chromosomes, which was not possible through conventional microscopic analysis. The technique at present relates to a rare form of intellectual disability, but the principle is likely to apply more broadly.[3] Virtual reality (VR) techniques are being developed to provided a quick and non-intrusive means to assess brain damage. It is safer to assess spatial cognition through a VR kitchen than in a real kitchen – a virtual pan of boiling water hurts no one.

One of the reasons for the lowering of 'safe' or threshold levels is improved assessment of exposure of individuals, but it has been difficult to demonstrate exposure within a time frame. Hair samples can achieve this – an alien substance at the ends was there before one at the roots – but data are clouded because it is necessary to take measurements only of a substance that has been fixed within hair from the roots outwards, and this can be contaminated by the same substance on the surface of the hair coming from elsewhere. New techniques using the nuclear probe microscope at the University of Oxford will overcome this problem. From looking at the core of hair sections it will be possible to measure the intake of heavy metals accurately over several years.[4]

There will also be improved understandings of the mechanisms of brain impairment. For example, research about fats has so far concentrated mainly on the unnecessary ones which constitute unhealthy, excess accumulations in overweight individuals. But there is relatively little work about the consequences of the absence of *necessary* fats that are crucial for healthy brain development. The former is a wealthy-nation concern – overeating – the latter is a poor-world concern – malnutrition – and so has been sidelined.

Another new perception stems from increased understandings of apoptosis – programmed cell death – which is a natural part of foetal development. Initially the foetus contains unnecessary cells (for example, webbing between fingers and toes) which are programmed to disappear at a certain point in development. The brain develops in much the same way, and it is possible that some environmental toxins may interfere with the programming, causing unnecessary cells to remain and necessary ones to die.

It might seem reasonable to assume that progress will be confined to developments in imaging or understanding of the brain and genetic material, and that improvements in the assessment of intelligence will either remain incremental or arise from changes in how we view intelligence. But this may not be so. At the Foetal Behaviour Centre at Queen's University, Belfast, Professor Peter Hepper and his team claim that they can now assess the mental ability of a foetus at about 24 weeks. The technique, habituation, involves testing the capacity to learn through monitoring responses to sound. A foetus should learn to ignore repeated sounds by remembering that they are unimportant – ignoring things that are irrelevant is a basic form of learning. The unborn child should also learn to recognize its mother's voice at 30 weeks. Testing intelligence before birth may improve the protective sciences, because in the womb there are far fewer confounding variables from the social environment which make assessment of intelligence after birth so problematic, such as parenting style and education.

The work at Belfast has a significance beyond the assessment of intelligence. It also suggests further ways in which the foetus may be vulnerable to environmental factors. If unborn children are starting to learn through using their auditory senses, what is the effect if a mother works or lives in a high-noise environment while pregnant? There is existing evidence that noise exposure relates to other developmental outcomes,[5] but it seems plausible that there will eventually be evidence that exposure to excessive noise before birth also affects the ability to learn.

Assessing the effect on the intellect will also embrace new conceptualizations, which go beyond the simple measurement of an impact on intelligence in a static time frame. This is indicated by current research at the EPA Neurotoxicology Division in North Carolina.[6] The WHO definition of intellectual disability embraces deficits both of IQ and of adaptive skills. Animal studies by the EPA's Robert MacPhail suggest that environmental toxins such as pesticides can affect these adaptive skills. He proposes that the brain may be more sensitive to chemical toxins in relation to our ability to adapt from one environmental challenge to the next than in relation to the more straightforward ability to intellectualize individual tasks. This threat is very important for both individual and human survival. In MacPhail's words:

> Adaptation to the environment is an evolutionary hallmark that ensures survival and perpetuation of a species, and a cardinal feature of the development of individual organisms throughout life. Deficits in the ability to adapt following exposure to environmental contaminants can have major consequences for the individual.

Recent human studies seem to support MacPhail's laboratory work. Helen Daly, director of the Center for Neurobehavioral Effects of Environmental Toxins in New York, has found a decline in the habituation skills of newborn babies around the area of the polluted Great Lakes. From work between 1991 and 1994, with hundreds of infants whose mothers had eaten fish contaminated with toxins such as PCBs and dioxin, she found that there was a 'clear and predictable' reduction in the ability of babies to adjust to irritants such as lights, rattles, bells and pokes.

We now live in a world in which we create environments that change with increasing rapidity, and at the same time create new chemical hazards that seem to reduce our ability to cope with that change. The effects on human adaptive skills may eventually become a far more important area of study than simple understandings of intellectual decline as a static entity.

## Risk assessment

Environmental risk assessment is now a major protector of human life and well-being – or at least it should be. Whether or not we are poisoned through food additives, chemicals in water supplies or toxins in the air depends upon an army of scientists who advise, with varying degrees of integrity, governments and industry. Risk assessment is less a question of 'to ban or not to ban', and more a matter of 'how much can we chance?' If modern risk assessment were clearly understood by the public, it might demand as much media attention as the police or the military. But, as yet, its role in human security is largely ignored.

> The new risks have produced a new breed of shamans, called risk assessors. As with the shamans and physicians of old, it might be more dangerous to go to them for advice than to suffer unattended [because of] the dangers of this new alchemy where body counting replaces social and cultural values and excludes us from participating in decisions about the risks that a few have decided the many cannot do without. The issue is not risk but power.[7]

A significant problem is the reliance on old, opportunistic data deriving from catastrophes which, it is hoped, will not be repeated, such as the Chisso mercury poisoning at Minamata Bay, Japan, in the 1950s and 1960s. Work with the Hiroshima and Nagasaki survivors still provides the principal reference point underpinning current 'safe' levels for radiation exposure. Dr Alice Stewart maintains that, because certain groups of people were excluded from the population originally studied, the results are very questionable, yet the error is now incorporated into risk estimates world-wide.[8] The Japanese victims suffered a single exposure. A worker in nuclear plant may suffer very low-level but ongoing exposure. Currently we rely on data derived from the first scenario to protect the individual faced with the second, yet to assume that the two are comparable may be incorrect.

Risk assessment in relation to EMID is likely to change significantly in the near future, but not necessarily in the direction of greater certainty. The results of experimental and observational science should in theory culminate in so-called safe or threshold levels upon which a risk assessment can be based. The idea that there is a lowest observed adverse effect level (LOAEL) or no observed adverse effect level (NOAEL) derives mainly from work in relation to health impacts that are reasonably clear, such as cancer. Even in this sphere the approach is far from conclusive, but it is much less helpful when the outcome is intellectual decline. The US National Research Council recently concluded that 'Commonly used paradigms for risk assessment do not accurately model the risks associated with exposure to neurotoxicants', and elaborated:

> The NOAEL–LOAEL approach is based on an assumption of a threshold, a dose below which an effect does not change in incidence or severity. However, the evidence of the general applicability of that assumption for all neurotoxicants is relatively weak. Even though a given neurological response may require a threshold dose of a specific toxicant, other toxicants in the environment that cause the same or similar response may in effect lower the threshold dose of the specific neurotoxic of interest. That is, a person may have a threshold of effect in a pure environment, but there may not be a threshold for a heterogeneous population in a heterogeneous environment. It is likely that some neurotoxicants have thresholds and others do not . . . the nervous system is composed of cells that are non-replaceable, which would argue that no damage can be considered innocuous . . . the application of the NOAEL–LOAEL approach to all neurotoxicants is unlikely to be biologically defensible.[9]

Risk assessment concerning radiation and cancer is now tending towards the 'linear, no-threshold hypothesis', i.e. any exposure poses a threat: there is no safe level of exposure. In 1980 the US National Academy of Sciences held that there was a safe level, but its BEIR V report of 1990 unanimously accepts the linear, no-threshold hypothesis, which is a major change in scientific opinion.[10] This is mirrored in relation to EMID. Evidence from the United Nations Scientific Committee on the Effects of Atomic Radiation (UNSCEAR) concerning intellectual decline caused by ionizing radiation has changed the view that there is a clear safe level of radiation exposure: 'Although the data do not suffice to define precisely the shape of the dose–effect curve, they imply that there may be little, if any, threshold for the effect when the brain is in its most sensitive stage of development.'[11]

Scientific opinion is clearly changing fast, but conclusions about the degree of risk posed by a particular agent are rarely framed in the light of *trends* of safe levels, yet this is perfectly possible. In 1988, UNSCEAR cautioned that 'risk estimates may need substantial revision downward (particularly in the low-dose ranges)'. By 1993, the prediction was considered correct.[12] Such candour is unusual, but acknowledging trends need not stop at a cautionary caveat. In her study of lead exposure among

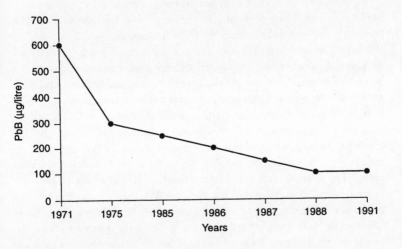

**Figure 4.1**   The evolution of lead critical limits, 1971–1991.
*Source:* Françoise Barten, *Environmental Lead Exposure of Children in Managua, Nicaragua: An Urban Health Problem* (CIP-Gegevens, Koninklijke Bibliotheek: The Hague, 1992). Reproduced with permission.

communities in Managua, Françoise Barten demonstrates that 'critical limit' trends can be presented in a more illuminating way than is normal (Figure 4.1). (Some studies now conclude that there 'is no evidence of a safe level' for lead.[13])

The presentation of this simple graph provides an indication of where safe levels might be going, and raises an obvious question. Why did those setting safe levels a few years ago not present this in the context of a downward trend? Had they done so, public opinion would have been better informed. If such a graph showed a bottoming-out or upward trend in recent assessments, it might be reasonable to conclude that the safe level was adequate. (But there seems to be not one instance of a safe threshold being raised because of new research.) A curve showing a steep downward trend would suggest that there is further to fall. Commercial decisions, risking billions of dollars, are based on simple graphs of this nature. So why is such an obvious form of presentation not adopted in science? Perhaps because 'safe level' assessments are commonly commissioned by governments, and the primary intention is probably that the results are safe for the government, not for the public.

'Safe' levels derive from calculations based on the vulnerability of a supposed 'average human'. Usually this means a theoretical model reflecting the white, Western, wealthy, healthy, well-housed, well-fed, adult male.

In experimental terms it usually means the white, healthy, well-housed, well-fed mouse. In a global context, the theoretical 'average human' is far from average – and sometimes far from human. Actual, as opposed to theoretical, human communities embody a variety of groups which may be especially vulnerable. In poorer countries most of the population is below the 'average' because of health problems and malnutrition, and these are usually the people at greatest risk from environmental threats.

Is the 'average' notion even credible in all circumstances? Gender affects vulnerability, and gender reflects *difference* – there is no 'average' gender. If females are more susceptible to a certain threat, but the 'safe' level reflects an average across males and females, all females are as a result less safe than males. The circumstance is far from hypothetical. For example, boys are more susceptible to fragile X syndrome. (Whereas females inherit two copies of the X chromosome, males inherit only one and so are more likely to suffer the full effects of a damaged copy.) There is evidence that the brains of female infants may be more vulnerable than those of males at some developmental stages, because various parts of the brain develop at different times in males and females and there is a consequent vulnerability to toxins that attack particular sites.[14]

It might appear possible to factor into assessments the high-risk groups such as 'infants', but it is not so simple in the field of EMID. While it is true that infants are much more susceptible to some threats, such as lead, in other circumstances the plasticity of the younger brain means that it can compensate partially for an injury that would result in much greater impairment in an adult.[15] In 1996, *New Scientist* reported a remarkable case of a 9-year-old boy who had only ever been able to say 'Mama'. For clinical reasons he had half his brain surgically removed, and he then learned to speak. This overturned previous theories that language acquisition could not take place after the age of 6.[16]

To account for a range of vulnerabilities, risk assessment techniques add an uncertainty factor, which is essentially an informed guess. Is this adequate? The UN SCOPE committee elaborates:

> *These [vulnerability] factors include developmental stages (e.g. the developing embryo, the aged), nutritional deficiencies, disease states, genetic conditions, behavioural factors, and previous or concomitant exposures . . . Present guidelines . . . from studies on the average animal or human include a 10-fold uncertainty factor . . . to extrapolate from the average to the sensitive human. However, the actual variability arising from the intrinsic and extrinsic factors listed above is not known.*[17]

Even this honest overview omits the cumulative and intergenerational aspect of EMID, which further emphasizes the shaky ground upon which the 'average human' approach to risk assessment is based. A recent study linking Down's syndrome to low-dose radiation, in the UK, found that the rate of the syndrome peaked at the time of high, whole-body radiation doses from fall-out from nuclear testing. In any population there is usually a higher level of Down's syndrome births among women over 35, but even when this was taken into account the peaks showed a far greater effect among older women, in one instance rocketing from 67 to 431 cases per 10,000 births. An explanation was proposed by the researcher Dr John Bound: 'It seems that the total dose you've had in your life is much more important than any individual dose. The greater susceptibility of older women suggests that these low doses may be the straw that broke the camel's back.'[18]

In this circumstance the vulnerability factors are gender, pregnancy, age (mid-life, *not* old age or infancy) and accumulated dose. And the outcome will not be detectable until the next, and possibly other future, generations. What is the answer to the child, born with Down's syndrome because of radiation, who asks, 'Why did risk assessment not protect me?' Only one response comes to mind: 'You chose the wrong mother.' And, once again, how does this all relate to those who have a pre-existing intellectual disability? Certainly they would fall into many of the standard 'vulnerability' categories. Take one example, phenylketonuria (PKU). This is a condition that, from birth, can create a severe intellectual disability unless the child is given a diet for five or six years that avoids phenylalanine, which PKU sufferers cannot metabolize fully and which will cause brain impairment. In the USA alone, around four million people suffer from PKU. The food sweetener aspartame, marketed as a substitute for saccharine, is now used widely in soft drinks. Phenylalanine is one of the main constituents of aspartame. There is a further intergenerational twist: raised phenylalanine levels in mothers can lead to intellectual disabilities in their babies.

In nations like the USA and UK it is at least possible to screen babies and inform the parents of children with PKU of the danger – although 'rather you than me' trying to keep any child away from soft drinks and other sweetened junk foods until the age of 6, with the pressures of current advertising. But what of the threat posed by the Cola Colonization of the poor countries, where the original condition may not even have been diagnosed in many children?

Does the effect of sweeteners stop neatly at the boundaries of current scientific knowledge? Professor Robert Wurtman of the Massachusetts Institute of Technology (MIT) presents his view very simply:

> *The quantity of aspartame in soft drinks causes brain levels of phenylalanine the like of which has never occurred in man's evolutionary history. It's going*

> *to be a fascinating experiment in brain chemistry. Do we really want to conduct this experiment?*[19]

Vulnerable individuals may turn out to be the miners' canaries – those who clearly demonstrate adverse effects which are less apparent, but still significant, in wider populations.

Aspartame has not been banned because of children with PKU, and this is a known, not theoretical, vulnerable group. We can decide to view people with specific vulnerabilities in one of two ways. Either they are 'sick', 'lucky to receive treatment', and must make the best of their 'disease'; or they are fully part of the human race. At present we accept that a vulnerability such as PKU morally sanctions a shift of responsibility from the poisoner to the victim.

Current risk assessment methods abandon the most vulnerable – conceptually, commonly through lack of data and sometimes deliberately. This highlights a stark difference between a scientific view of risk, which works on the basis of the vulnerability of a theoretical 'average human', and a human rights view, which derives from a baseline representing the protection of the *most* vulnerable. Among the most vulnerable to neurotoxins are people with a pre-existing intellectual disability, not least because of their susceptibility to the synergistic effects caused by inherent micro-nutrient deficiencies and unpredictable behaviour. This means that at least 3 per cent of any population is absent from current conceptualizations within all spheres of the protective sciences and risk assessment. Yet the necessary scientific evidence is commonly available.

It is misleading to focus entirely on the vagaries of scientific method. The human factor is sometimes a greater determinate of actual, as opposed to theoretical, risk faced by a population. In 1985 the UK government tested the efficiency of checking food for lead and cadmium across 40 of its analytical laboratories.[20] Of the 25 that returned results (!), only three were within the limits of accuracy set by official standards. The government scientists who conducted the survey felt that the results were 'certainly no worse than results from similar international schemes'. Time does not seem to improve things. In 1995, the UK Secretary for the Environment complained that results concerning identical water samples sent to analytical laboratories in each member state in the EU varied by a factor of up to 1000.[21]

Risk assessment assumes that relevant human expertise is at least located in the right places. This is not always so. A US Congress report concludes of priorities in America, 'An agency's approach to neurotoxicity evaluation often corresponds to the presence or absence of neurotoxicologists on staff', and quotes the Office of Technology and Assessment, which believes that 'effectiveness in addressing neurotoxicological concerns at Federal agencies is dependent on the presence of neurotoxicologists in regulating programme offices'.[22]

These examples come from state-of-the-art wealthy nations. What is the position in poorer countries, where scarce resources, bribery and lack of professional expertise can compound the human factor infinitely? And how, if at all, do these crucial human factors get incorporated into formal risk assessment?

Within current risk assessment practice, if data are lacking or inadequate the default mode is that a potential threat is rarely declared unsafe. For example, it is established that mercury is a potential neurotoxin and that the foetus generally is at greater risk than the mother. From existing research, the risk to the foetus at a certain level of exposure might be given as one in so many thousand births. But as there is no conclusive research about the effects of mercury on the ova of a female foetus, this possible threat to a pregnant woman's grandchild will probably be ignored, even though ova are possibly more vulnerable than the female foetus they are within.

Put this approach another way. If you are given a revolver and told that it has one bullet, you know the odds for Russian roulette – the 'risk assessment'. But what if you do not know whether or not the revolver is loaded? It might have six bullets or it might have none. In the first scenario 'risk assessment' puts the chance of death as one in six. In the second scenario, if you apply current principles, something *called* 'risk assessment' would probably deem the gun not dangerous.

## Intergenerational eugenics

Largely missing from the current 'intergenerational justice' debate is the question, unjust to exactly whom? Is it future generations as a whole who will suffer the adverse consequences of environmental change, or specific groups within future generations? Intuitively, the response might be that 'the weakest' of future generations will suffer, but how true is this? What is the possibility and probable pattern of intergenerational EMID?

Parent–child genetic transfer is beyond dispute, and a direct inherited effect two generations hence is very possible because a woman's eggs are formed when she is a foetus and if damaged may not recover. The exposure of a pregnant woman to a toxic substance or radiation today could affect the brains of her children or grandchildren. The persistent hormone-disrupting chemicals present a similar short-term intergenerational hazard (see Appendix).

The long-term argument is that adverse germ-line changes, arising from environmental exposures, could be passed down infinitely through generations until intellectual and health status is so poor that those family lines eventually die out. This seems improbable on the basis of data from the Japanese survivors of the US A-bombs, but not impossible. More recent research following the nuclear power disaster at Chernobyl has found increased germ-line mutations in children 290 kilometres from the reactor.[23] From recent understandings of one of the intrinsic causes of intellectual disability, fragile X, the epidemiologist Tom Fryers hints that isolated intergenerational effects, of environmental origin, might already occur. He asks, 'Could there have been some widespread environmental insult many generations ago which gave rise to multiple mutations that are still affecting populations of European origin?'[24] In a few instances, it may now be too late to put right the effects of environmental mistakes for any generation.

But it is not necessary to enter the realms of science fiction and germ-line mutation to predict intergenerational effects. In poorer regions, the same family lineages will probably be subject to the same industrial toxins, the same micro-nutrient deficiencies and the same interrelated poverty–health–nutrition spirals. The inheritance of intellectual potential is chemical *and* social.

This simple, social intergenerational effect is compounded by an obvious human factor. Like it or not, intelligence is a determining aspect in finding a life partner, in societies where marriages are arranged and in societies where they are not. (In the words of one Indian broker, 'A degree is worth a hundred cows.') So those suffering intellectual decline will inevitably gravitate towards one another and intensify any environmentally precipitated genetic changes through consanguineous genetic inheritance, and, unless effectively supported, perpetuate a degenerative psycho-social environment. In the context of the poorer countries, such family lines may not survive long.

Since the A-bombs, scientists have been consumed with exploring the possibility of germ-line genetic inheritance, and this has obscured the more probable consequences of social inheritance, which may or may not embrace somatic or germ-line effects. We have already set in motion a form of intergenerational eugenics, and it does not need a microscope to see it.

For millions of years, humans have evolved through optimum survival within the natural environment of our planet. Current human-made environmental change can threaten long-term human survival, but can also positively enhance it. Risk assessment should be the means to ensure that we err towards the latter. It should prevent intergenerational eugenics, yet it can be seen to precipitate the process. If safety within our new human-made global environment is based on the vulnerability of the 'average human', it follows that some groups of 'the weakest' will probably not survive prevailing and future environmental threats. This is questionable in itself, but viewed from a clinical perspective theoretically over infinite time it raises two other worrying aspects.

First, the elimination of the weakest might lead to a revision *upwards* of the notion of 'average human' vulnerability (otherwise it would no longer represent the average). Consequently the safe levels would become *less* strict, and in turn a new cadre of the most vulnerable would be created and then eliminated. In theory, over a very long time period this leads to the near extinction of the human race, because the 'average human' upon which safe levels are based would forever be moving upward as those at the bottom were eliminated. There is a balancing argument, that we would constantly be replenishing those who were eliminated by new cadres made vulnerable by the increasingly hazardous environmental mess, so the 'average human' would not be upwardly mobile. But either way we are reminded that the 'average human' is a marker constructed in relation to the human brain in a particular environment at a particular point in time – not an objective reference point that intrinsically protects us.

Second, it is often easiest to observe an adverse health effect in 'the weakest', which may have a less obvious effect throughout a population generally. Those with asthma are the first to indicate poor air quality; people with Down's syndrome or autism appear more sensitive to micro-nutrient deficiencies; PKU sufferers react visibly to phenylalanine-based food sweeteners. They act as the miner's canary – as human indicators of a potential human hazard. Put more starkly, from an environmental health standpoint the weakest serve a very useful protective function within any population, and if they are slowly eliminated everyone else becomes less safe.

Hopefully, these infinite-time scenarios are essentially science fiction. But it is less important to argue about exact outcomes than to look at the question that the argument raises. Why do we rely on risk assessment methods based on the 'average human', which are intended to ensure human survival, but which, when viewed theoretically over infinite time, have an inherent tendency to threaten that survival?

The solution is to avoid an assessment of risk that derives from notions of an 'average human' vulnerability, and replace this with a baseline that reflects what is known or theorized about the *most* vulnerable human groups. This is not science fiction – it reflects how medical drugs are tested, regulated and used. Injury of those who are vulnerable, by medicines, usually stems from a lack of scientific knowledge – not because injury of the most vulnerable is seen as a risk worth taking. Why is there a difference between risk assessment in relation to drugs and that relating to environmental toxins? In part because it is easy to establish causation and make drugs companies and governments accountable for injury to individuals. This is currently not so straightforward in relation to environmental hazards.

To reiterate the words of the US National Research Council, 'the nervous system is composed of cells that are non-replaceable, which would argue that no damage can be considered innocuous'.[25] Those who view the '*most* vulnerable human' approach as fundamentalist might stop to consider that this means vulnerable human *groups*, not isolated individuals with rare health conditions, and that even this approach will still leave a 'safe' level below which many will remain at significant risk. But their circumstance would not stem from the scientifically flawed and ethically questionable notion of average vulnerability. It would mark the divide between vulnerability that can be predicted, and vulnerability that cannot because of inadequate scientific knowledge, human failing and the environmental threats and synergisms that science cannot comprehend and probably never will even within a precautionary principle.

## Will scientific progress destroy the evidence of the problems it causes?

Scientific progress is a *cause* leading to a *problem*. It is also undeniably part of the *cure*. The dialogue between environmentalists and their adversaries rarely goes beyond arguing which of these perspectives has the greatest credibility.

But understanding the unique problems of relating the protective sciences to EMID brings up a third and more concerning aspect. Taken together, *cause*, *problem* and *cure* are all increasing exponentially, and this has the potential to *decrease* protective knowledge – the ability to monitor the nature and severity of the threats. At first this seems counter-intuitive. Figure 4.2 puts the argument in diagrammatic form.

### Increased cause

The increase of *cause* will present growing difficulties for research, not least, as the conclusions about toxicology suggest, in keeping pace with the scale of the chemical hazards. In particular, the increasing socio-biological synergisms, combining problems of *absence* and *presence*, will make assessment of adverse health outcomes increasingly difficult. In her Managuan study, Françoise Barten was presented with difficulties in establishing the dose–response relationship concerning lead take-up because many children also suffered iron deficiency, which precipitates lead absorption.[26] The more mixed up the environmental threats become, the greater the problems of assessing the effect of single agents.

The difficulties of identifying and measuring EMID in those with a pre-existing intellectual disability might seem minor statistically, given normal prevalence rates (3 per cent), but if prevalence escalates, studies that ignore this problem may become seriously flawed. In a community already suffering

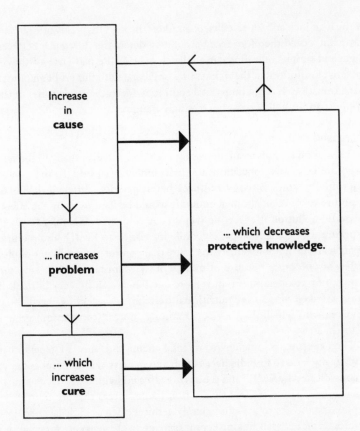

**Figure 4.2** The cause–problem–cure dynamic.

a 20 per cent prevalence of intellectual decline because of iodine deficiency, how do you start to assess the effects of a polluting lead smelter on intellectual abilities?

The contamination of samples and laboratory equipment, because of total contamination in the environment, is already a well-known problem. If a scientist needs to compare a sample that has been exposed to an environmental agent against a sample that has not been exposed, laboratories contaminated with the same agent will mask the difference. In 1981, work by a Californian geochemist, Clair Patterson, found that prevailing assessments of the current levels of environmental lead as compared to those in prehistoric samples were inaccurate by a factor of many hundreds. The reason: samples from polar ice used by previous researchers became contaminated in the laboratory, giving the impression that levels were also high in prehistoric times. Because Patterson's laboratory was plastic-lined, with an air lock and super-efficient air filters, he kept his prehistoric samples clean and could therefore more accurately detect the difference between them and samples reflecting current levels of lead.[27] Perhaps state-of-the-art research institutions in the rich nations will cope with this problem of total contamination, but the more vital routine work in the laboratories of the poorer nations will become increasingly fraught.

## Increased problem

Increasing cause leads to an increasing problem, and eventually to the *total* exposure of whole populations to environmental hazards. To make valid assessments, epidemiology requires heterogeneity: differing levels of exposure to a potential causal entity. It would be hard to study the effects of traffic pollution if everyone were to be subjected to similar levels of exposure. But epidemiology, especially in relation to EMID, also requires a parallel level of homogeneity to ensure that control groups do not display different outcomes because of extraneous circumstances. Assessing the impact of a toxic exposure in remote rural areas can be very difficult if those affected also suffer nutritional deficiencies affecting intellectual development, which may not occur among control (comparison) groups in urban areas.

The exposure to some environmental chemicals is now so general that it is already hard to find the necessary heterogeneity within homogeneity: groups affected by EMID and groups not affected, within otherwise similar populations. There are few rich-nation communities that are not totally exposed to the oestrogen-mimicking chemicals such as phthalates, so epidemiological research linking sperm damage to these agents is becoming more difficult. Nearly all babies in the rich nations have now been subjected to ultrasound scans, so further investigation of the suspicion that scans might affect learning ability is virtually impossible. Are there enough rich-nation children who have not ingested phenylalanine from drinks sweeteners to provide a control group if scientists in the future decide to investigate further the impact of this chemical? The possibilities of creating protective knowledge decrease as the problem increases and exposure becomes total.

Unthinking politicians occasionally complain along the lines that 'half of our schoolchildren have below average scores'. However good or bad the school system, in any corner of the world, half the children will always be below the average. Otherwise, it would not be the average. But the mistake prompts a crucial reminder: average intelligence is a floating concept.

IQ scores are calculated in relation to an average (IQ 100). If intellectual decline affects whole populations, the average must eventually be lowered (in relation to objective, or 'criterion-referenced', standards), as otherwise statistical method will fail for assessments within those populations. The result would be a new subjective ('norm-referenced') average: IQ 100 would mean a lower level of ability by objective standards. So, at least in theory, over an infinite time period, total intellectual decline in a whole population could be significant but IQ tests would not measure this. If everyone in a community suffers intellectual decline, no one does.

Because of cultural difference and the predominance of Western methods, we are still trying to determine what 'IQ 100' means for much of the global population. When and if this is determined, will it be the true average of human intellectual potential within a particular culture, or an average reflecting intellectual abilities that have already declined from the optimum because of environmental factors? In African cities, where 90 per cent of children now have blood lead levels that affect intellectual ability, and nutritional problems, the scenario is not just theoretical.

## Increased cure

The increase of cure, in the form of better medical diagnoses and treatment, may also decrease protective knowledge over a long time scale. There are already isolated examples. In a widely researched case of methylmercury poisoning through contaminated grain in Iraq in 1971–2, researchers experienced problems with their data because victims with the most conspicuous symptoms sought treatment sooner than those who had suffered lower levels of exposure. As a consequence the usual dose–response pattern – the greater the dose the more serious the effect – was less clear. Scientific progress in the form of medical cure had intervened, clouding the evidence of cause and effect.

In the Iraq case the chemical was well known and the exposed population big enough for useful data still to be collected, even with confused evidence at the serious end of exposure. But if the chemical is new and unknown, and the exposed population small, cure can confound *any* useful research, and the outcome in terms of public protection is cause for concern. In 1973, particular spray adhesives were banned in the USA following experimental work linking industrial exposure of women to chromosome breaks and birth defects. As a result of knowing the possible risk, nine women had abortions. But the women's pre-emptive actions also meant that it was not possible for further human studies to confirm the preliminary findings. Because of this lack of evidence, the ban on the use of the substance was lifted six months later.[28]

The science of detecting foetal impairments is well-funded and fast-moving because of the perceived high cost, to the state, of caring for severely disabled people. A few years ago it was not possible to screen pregnant women for the possibility of Down's syndrome in their unborn children. Now amniocentesis is common throughout the world, effective at 16 weeks of pregnancy. But a much simpler technique developed by the UK company Applied Imaging may well soon replace amniocentesis. The test is based on a sample of the mother's blood, analysed by computerized imaging techniques, and is effective as early as 12, perhaps 10, weeks. Here again, cure will diminish the possibilities for research about risk. There is little chance of assessing brain impairment in aborted foetuses, even if the resources were made available to try.

As the nuclear industry disaster at Chernobyl demonstrated, pregnant women who believe that their children might be impaired in the womb by an environmental impact will often opt for abortions. So these fast-improving screening techniques could eliminate many birth problems caused by an exposure to an agent that is thought to be a reproductive hazard – for example, from an explosion at a chemical factory which releases a chemical about which little is known, as at Bhopal. Scientific progress in the form of better screening and the termination of births might be seen as a benefit to a community in this circumstance, but it also removes the evidence needed to prove that the agent is a threat and to argue for measures to prevent similar exposures. Research following disasters is still a main source of evidence about environmental threats.

There is another twist to the cure perspective. In some circumstances the nature of the cause can be established only *after* some form of preventive, social cure has been implemented. Before the introduction of unleaded petrol in the UK and USA, the leaded petrol industry maintained that petrol was not the source of the elevated levels of lead known to exist in children's bodies. It was only a few years after the introduction of unleaded petrol, when lead levels in children had reduced dramatically, that the direct link with leaded petrol could be proved. In the USA, a 55 per cent reduction of lead in petrol caused a 37 per cent reduction in blood lead levels in a sample of one million. We often need to stop polluting to show that we need to stop polluting – to stop a cause to prove a cause.

## The cause–problem–cure dynamic
It seems that over an infinite time period, the increase of cause creates a increase in problem and also an increase in the response: medical and social cure. As an outcome of the increase of each, the efficacy of the main re-straining influence on increasing cause – protective knowledge – decreases. If we view this in relation to the main question of *Terminus Brain* – are the small-scale instances of EMID indicative of something larger – we are presented with an uncomfortable conclusion. Over a very long time period, the dynamics are such that it may be scientifically impossible to detect large-scale effects. And remember that the starting-point, the basic research to prove causal links in small communities, is itself extremely problematic.

## When science fails

The Mad Hatter in *Alice in Wonderland* did not derive entirely from Lewis Carroll's imagination. He was a parody of a nineteenth-century phenomenon. Many hatters really were mad, because of the use of mercury in the process of hat-making. It did not need scientific method to create a public awareness of this problem – 'as mad as a hatter' was a common phrase at this time. During the same period, the decision to prohibit the employment of young women in the lead factories arose from a simple observation: their children were being born with too many noticeable disabilities.

The question this poses is not how people knew that mercury or lead was the cause of a health problem without modern science. The answer to this is self-evident: observation and common sense. The question is why it took so long for the most technically advanced nation in the world to respond to occupational health problems that Hippocrates had noted in 400 BC concerning lead, and those operating the mercury mines in Almader in Spain have recognized for 2400 years.

Science may be limited, but we can still build viable survival strategies based on a combination of limited scientific knowledge, general observation and common-sense application of resultant beliefs. The next three chapters are therefore of no less significance because they describe a social model of cause and effect. Social understandings help to develop a balanced common-sense perception which, because most of the global population lives more within the problem side of scientific progress than that of cure or cause, may have more relevance for human survival for them than the fine-tuning of scientific understandings.

---

## Notes

1. A.W. Macara, 'Lead pollution: report of the Welsh Community Medicine Conference', *Newsletter of the Faculty of Community Medicine* (April 1976), p. 1.

2. Tom Fryers, 'Epidemiological research related to mental retardation', *Current Opinion in Psychiatry* (1993), **6**(5), 650–5.

3. J. Flint, A.O.M. Wilkie, V.J. Buckle, R.M. Winter, A.J. Holland and H.E. McDermid, 'The detection of subtelomeric chromosome rearrangements in idiopathic mental retardation', *Nature Genetics* (1995), **9**, 132–40.

4. Julie Johnson, 'Probe overcomes hairy problem', *New Scientist* (1995), **1971**, 23.

5. Howard Hu and Mitchell Besser, 'Atmosphere variations, noise, and vibration', in Maureen Paul (ed.), *Occupational and Environmental Reproductive Hazards: A Guide for Clinicians* (Williams & Wilkins: Baltimore, 1993), pp. 218–32.

6. R.C. MacPhail, 'Neurotoxicology of adaptive behaviour', Neurotoxicology Division, Health Effects Research Laboratory, Office of Health Research Work Report (EPA: North Carolina Research Triangle, 1995).

7. Charles Perrow, *Normal Accidents: Living with High-Risk Technologies* (Basic Books: New York, 1984), p. 12.

8. Jill Sutcliffe and David Sumner, 'Low level radiation and health', *Global Security* (1995), **12**, 7.

9. NRC, *Environmental Neurotoxicology* (National Academy Press: Washington, DC, 1992), pp. 115–16.

10. Eric Chivian *et al.*, *Critical Condition: Human Health and the Environment* (MIT Press: Cambridge, MA, 1993), p. 96.

11. NRC, *Health Effects of Exposure to Low Levels of Ionizing Radiation* (BEIR V) (National Academic Press: Washington, DC, 1990), p. 7.

12. UNSCEAR, *Sources and Effects of Ionizing Radiation* (United Nations: New York, 1993), p. 806.

13. M. Fulton *et al.*, 'Influence of blood lead on the ability and attainment of children in Edinburgh', *The Lancet*, 30 May 1987.

14. R.W. Thatcher, R.A. Walker and S. Giudice, 'Human cerebral hemispheres develop at different rates and ages', *Science* (1987), **236**, 1110–13.

15. M.E. Goldberger and M. Murray, 'Recovery of function and anatomical plasticity after damage to the adult and neonatal spinal cord', in C.W. Cotman (ed.), *Synaptic Plasticity* (Guilford Press: New York, 1985), pp. 77–110.

16. Alison Motluk, 'When half a brain is better than one', *New Scientist*, 20 April 1996, **2026**, p. 16.

17. V.B. Vouk and P.J. Sheenhan, *Methods for Assessing the Effects of Mixtures of Chemicals* (John Wiley & Sons: New York, 1987), pp. 736–7.

18. Owen Dyer, 'Study links low dose radiation and Down's syndrome', *British Medical Journal* (1995), **310**, 1088–9. Full report in *Journal of Epidemiology and Community Health* (1995), **49**, 164–70.

19. John Elkinton, *The Poisoned Womb* (Penguin Books: Harmondsworth, 1986), p. 229.

20. Royal Society of Chemistry, *Chemistry in Britain*, (1985), **11**.

21. 'Quarter of tap water fails to pass pesticide test', *Guardian*, 25 November 1995, p. 5.

22. US Congress/OTA, *Neurotoxicology: Identifying and Controlling Poisons of the Nervous System*, OTA-BA-436 (Government Printing Office: Washington, DC, 1990), p. 19.

23. Douglas Holdstock, 'Health effects of low-level radiation', *Global Security* (1996), **14**, 8.

24. Tom Fryers, 'Recent research in epidemiology', *Current Opinion in Psychology* (1993), **6**(5), 643–8.

25. NRC, *op. cit.* (n. 9).

26. Françoise Barten, *Environmental Lead Exposure of Children in Managua, Nicaragua* (CIP-Gegevens Koninklijke Bibliotheek: The Hague, 1992).

27. Des Wilson, *The Lead Scandal* (Heinemann: London, 1983), p. 43.

28. E.B. Hook and K.M. Healey, Untitled, *Science* (1976), **191**, 566–7.

# PART III

# The Social Environment

---

# CHAPTER 5

# Bounded Threats: Home and Work

---

Lead does not 'cause brain damage' – it is the way in which we choose to use lead that poses the threat. The cause of EMID is how local and global communities organize themselves – environmental agents are simply the potential cause. It is therefore crucial to develop an understanding of the social dynamics of an environmental threat, because these are probably more amenable to change than are chemicals or human biology.

The earliest understandings of EMID stem from the 'bounded' environments of home (in the broad sense of 'where you live') and workplace, because in these settings causation is easiest to observe and establish, and prevention, regulation and remediation might be implemented with relative ease. But the boundaries usually stem from rich-nation perceptions. In poorer countries, the divides are less distinct. Challenging these rich-nation perceptions is crucial because they still underpin environmental regulation and research in poorer nations, making it irrelevant to the lives of much of the population in those countries.

## Home

Home should provide security, sanctuary and respite from the perils of the outside world. But in relation to environmental hazards, this is not always the case. The problem is less the increasing scale of potential hazards, and more that the individual patterns of people's daily lives are rarely fully accounted for in the assessment of risk. Homes are houses plus humans, not just buildings.

The increased use of toxic substances in building materials and consumer goods is clearly problematic. Vapours from sealants, glues, particle boards, paints and domestic cleaners are often mildly neurotoxic. Pesticides are used in greater amounts in some American suburbs than in agricultural regions. Although the general risk is probably minimal, it increases significantly for those in the family who enjoy DIY or gardening, or do all the cleaning.

Even standard household fittings are not without some risk. A low level of carbon monoxide (CO) poisoning from gas water-heaters and fires is linked to an immediate slowing of brain function; at 'mild but chronic' levels of exposure, to foetal brain damage and other impairments.[1] Serious CO poisoning, if it does not kill, generally causes permanent brain impairment.

The safety of mobile phones is in question. From experiments on rats, Henry Lai and N. P. Singh of the University of Washington in Seattle believe that microwave radiation causes hot spots in the brain which can damage the DNA in brain cells. Thirty per cent of the energy radiating from the aerial is absorbed by the brain of the user. Use in a car intensifies the electromagnetic field. Standards for microwave exposure in the former Soviet Union were far stricter than those in the West. Was this because of the absence of commercial lobbying?

Cumulative and synergistic effects arising from personal habit are probably more significant than single threats. Aluminium cooking pots may seem harmless, but not in circumstances such as in India, where certain acidic food additives seem to dissolve the aluminium and the situation is worsened by the common practice of scouring with wire wool. Add to this the high levels of aluminium sometimes found in Indian instant coffee and the intake, which is linked to dementia and memory problems, can be significant.[2]

Innovations can pose a hazard because they are used in unexpected ways. Aluminium boil-in-the-bag food packages became a problem in the Canadian army two decades ago because, although they were lined with plastic to prevent direct contamination, soldiers often used the unprotected side of the bag as a plate and the water in which the bags had been boiled to make hot drinks.

The lesson from these two examples stems from the difference between home in the form of countless numbers of private dwellings, each with a differing range of hazards and unique patterns of human behaviour, and home in the form of a nation's army camps, in which a whole cadre of human beings face similar hazards and are generally behaving in much the same way.

The health effects of aluminium became evident in the Canadian military because everyone was exposed to the same threat; the effects were therefore widespread and conspicuous, medical monitoring of everyone was ongoing irrespective of the specific hazard and habits were similar and could easily be observed. Most importantly, the responsible entity had a vested interest in the prevention of intellectual dysfunction and poor health. This is not so in most domestic settings, and the difference emphasizes the problem of identifying and then preventing environmental hazards in the normal home. The risk of aluminium poisoning to Canadian soldiers was minor but quickly corrected, while countless Indians apparently continue to poison themselves to an unquantified degree with their coffee, curries and cooking pots.

It is misleading to conclude that all the hazards are of recent origin. From Roman times the problems caused by lead used in building materials – paint, water pipes, water tanks, putty – have been observed, hyped and forgotten. A Scottish study in relation to lead in tap water, in the1970s, found that women who drank contaminated water were twice as likely to have babies who were mentally retarded.[3] The hazard from lead in ceramic glazes, crystal, solder in food cans or newsprint is well known, although not usually considered substantial. Lead paint on toys has still not been banned in every country, and although toys commercially imported to nations with strict controls are screened, there is no protection against gifts or informal importing for resale by individuals.

Researchers from the University of North Carolina found in 1990 that the water supply in about a quarter of American homes contains 'dangerously high' concentrations of lead.[4] A 1993 report from the UK National Children's Bureau rediscovered the problem in Britain, but the British government has been slow to respond, perhaps because even back in the 1980s the cost of preventing exposure from just one source, drinking water, was put at over £1 billion. More than 10 per cent of UK homes have lead levels in drinking water which exceed the WHO safe level. In Blackburn, Lancashire, levels can sometimes be more than 1000 times the EU limit, because the local water dissolves the lead pipes very easily. In 1992, the USA suddenly demonstrated a specific concern with lead from ageing solder in water pipes.[5] A year later the UK government *abandoned* plans for abolishing the use of lead solder in pipes.

Again, personal habit plays its part. If mother is always up first in the morning, making herself a wake-up cup of tea, she is likely to take in more lead from old pipework than other family members, because the greatest risk comes when water has been sitting in the pipes for more than six hours. American environmental health lecturers tell their students the story of a wealthy New Yorker who suffered significant neurological problems which went undiagnosed for many years. The reason was a nineteenth-century family heirloom – the lead glaze of her favourite tea-cup.

Lead is ubiquitous. Garden soil is commonly contaminated by lead from petrol and industrial sources. In old buildings the lead is reasonably inert and although paint chips eaten by children can appear to pose a major potential threat, they usually cause only minor increases in blood lead because the lead is sealed by other substances in the paint. The greatest hazard arises when old houses are renovated, demolished or damaged through fire, because inert forms are converted into fine particles which are easily distributed and absorbed. This poses a conundrum for those trying to reduce the hazard, because remedial work which solves a domestic problem can often make things worse for a community.

Lead is a well known and widespread environmental hazard, and to increase the threat seems inexcusable. Why, for example, in the 1980s were new housing estates built on the former sites of old gasworks that were known to be toxic, in the London borough of Greenwich? Play areas at the development exposed children to extremely high levels of lead: 20,000 parts per million.

As leisure activities become more sophisticated, some replicating industrial processes on a small scale, a new range of hazards is created. Making ceramics at home causes exposure to heavy metals far exceeding that from simply using ceramic vessels. Art work, DIY and screen printing expose people to a range of neurotoxic solvents.[6] Often the keen amateur will take risks that would be banned in a commercial setting, such as working with poor ventilation.

Other contemporary forms of recreation can create less obvious non-chemical hazards for children. A UK study, by Dr Sally Ward of the Central Manchester Healthcare Trust, links noise from televisions, videos and hi-fi with delays in language development in young children. Babies exposed to high background noise ignored human voices, so cutting themselves off from early learning. Dr Ward reported 'horrifying noise levels . . . very loud tellies on constantly . . . three-month-olds propped in front of videos, older ones with headphones and story tapes. It seems to be a quite significant environmental change.'[7] Other studies relate home noise to lower ratings in creativity, spelling and language achievement. This situation is often compounded by noise from elsewhere: roads and airports. Although children adapt to noise levels this seems to be at the expense of cognitive skills.[8]

Recreation extends beyond the home, and new pastimes bring new problems, sometimes because of sub-standard equipment. Research among amateur scuba divers finds that those who dive more than forty times a year are likely to suffer intellectual decline. Small blood vessels in the central nervous system become obstructed by micro-bubbles that occur during decompression. Professional divers do not suffer similarly because they breathe a mix of helium and oxygen, not just compressed air, and they usually enjoy the protection of occupational health regulation.

Other wealthy pursuits are problematic: for example, the use of lead shot. Game birds are usually eaten after being cooked with the shot still in them. The total deposition of lead shot into the Canadian environment by waterfowl and other hunters is about 1500 to 2000 tonnes per year.[9]

In North America, recreational fishing has become problematic because of mercury levels in freshwater fish. The catch is commonly eaten, representing 20 per cent of US fish consumption, and, unlike with food

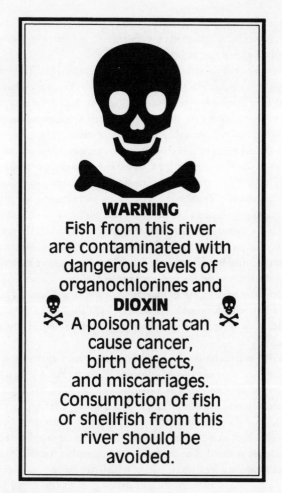

**Figure 5.1** Florida fishing warning.

in the shops, health hazards are not monitored.[10] Warnings are now common, but are probably more for the protection of the water authorities than the public (Figure 5.1).

There are three interesting aspects to recreational hazards. First, again, specific forms of human behaviour confound the intent of regulation based on the increasingly unworkable belief that environmental hazards respect convenient boundaries and that all human beings behave in accord with predictable norms. Second, the high level of publicity given to recreational hazards does not reflect their relative importance when compared with industrial pollution – but probably does reflect a political desire to shift public interest away from industry. And third, in the light of the scale of poor-nation problems, are scuba divers, mobile phones, game-hunters and anglers truly a global research priority?

The non-Western household poses different problems. The widespread use of naphthalene mothballs in countries such as Singapore has created a hazard. When combined with a specific enzyme deficiency at birth, prevalent in East Asia, mothballs cause neonatal jaundice and the possibility of resultant mental subnormality[11] (another *absence–presence* synergism).

In some Asian communities the use of cosmetics based on lead – khohl and surina – is another unique form of exposure to the metal through skin absorption. In Mexico, traditional ceramic manufacturing techniques create hazardous products.[12] Traditional pots – *jarro* and *casuele* – are glazed with lead oxide and continue to be used for cooking beans, rice and soup. But there is a tendency for Western medicine to overemphasize the more exotic causes of health problems in other countries – not all non-Western hazards are so obscure. Professor Tao Kuo-Tai of Nanjing University tells how, in Tibet, a common reason for brain injury in children is them falling from a particularly precarious form of staircase in traditional houses. The staircase is simply a log with footholds cut in it. There should be no assumption that tradition is inherently safe and the modern world always more hazardous.

From a Western outlook, such circumstances may appear easy to avoid because they seem so obviously cultural. But the lesson is that the same might be concluded of many rich-nation causes. Men from poor fishing communities, who dive for coral to earn a meagre living, risking brain impairment, would certainly wonder why wealthy scuba divers voluntarily expose themselves to the same hazard. Excessive car use for recreational reasons is clearly cultural. The impression commonly promoted is that non-Western customs are incidental habits which are simple to stop, and that Western customs are an intrinsic and major part of the social fabric and therefore impossible to change. If anything, the reverse is probably true.

In poorer dwellings the problems increase exponentially. A walk around any town in a poor nation at dusk brings with it the stench of kerosene lamps and cooking stoves. The fuel is usually leaded, although, when not used in vehicles, the lead serves no purpose. Charcoal braziers produce carbon monoxide at levels far exceeding general exposures from domestic gas fires (see above). Inevitably these fuels are used in enclosed spaces where children live, eat and sleep, and it is the women and girls who spend the most time in proximity to cooking stoves.

Water and food are commonly stored in containers that originally held toxic chemicals, the residues of which never disappear completely. In poor homesteads, old car-battery cases are now becoming a major domestic commodity. If UNICEF had to invent a flexible, all-purpose domestic resource it could do little better. Battery cases are used for seats, tables, larders, toys, building blocks and beds, and then burned as fuel for cooking and heating. Ingestion of battery ash is now one of the most significant sources of high levels of toxins in children.

It is when home and workplace are one, a common situation in poorer regions, that the Western perceptions become least relevant. Françoise Barten's superb study in Managua documents the conditions in the 200 *talleres artesanales de batería* – the cottage-based lead industry.[13] One-room dwellings, 4 metres square, are used for smelting, repairing and storing batteries, but also for cooking, eating and sleeping by the whole family. Food is often grown in polluted soil around the cottages.

In rural homesteads the dynamics become even less obvious. If fuel and water are becoming scarce because of environmental degradation, increasing time spent fetching these crucial resources reduces the time spent cultivating the land. As a consequence nutritional problems increase. In a poor home the threats come from every direction. This aspect is often missed in medical research, based on rich-nation perceptions, which generally relates to one hazard and one specific form of human behaviour within a Western stereotyped view of 'home'.

'Home' conjures up a picture of a child within a family, but this is now not the case for many children. Our understanding must extend to the orphanages, remand schools, prisons, non-governmental organization projects and urban streets which are home to millions. Institutions are often very far from stimulating or nurturing – they often cause an intellectual disability in otherwise unimpaired children. Media images of intellectually disabled children in orphanages in the former Soviet bloc and China largely depict children who are institutionalized because they are abandoned or have a minor learning difficulty, not because they initially had a significant disability.

## Work

The work environment has received considerable attention from researchers, particularly concerning reproductive hazards.[14] In the USA, concern culminated in the so-called 'foetal protection policies' in the 1970s. These did not always lead to cleaner workplaces, but often to women being denied work opportunities in potentially hazardous settings. In some cases employers demanded certificates of sterilization before they would employ younger women. The women's movement was quick to respond, not least by pointing out that reproductive hazards are also transmitted through men, and therefore policies aimed only at women were discriminatory. The main argument was that the workplace should be safe for everyone irrespective of reproductive status. This might make sense in richer nations, but the problems are certainly not resolved in poorer nations, where pressures to take employment, whatever the conditions, are overriding.

While reproductive hazards have received attention for many years, less obvious intellectual dysfunctions suffered by workers themselves are a more recent concern. In heavy industry, production involving manganese, for example, exposes workers (predominantly male) to dust from crushing processes and fumes from furnace tapping and cooling. Those experiencing even low-level exposure are known to suffer a decline in cognitive flexibility and motor functions.[15]

The microelectronics industry seems a particular culprit, because the industrial infrastructure is minimal and robust and the product is easily transportable, so factories can follow the most vulnerable labour supply, usually women. New organic solvents in paints, adhesives and glues are a significant problem. These can cause direct intellectual dysfunctions, such as memory loss and concentration difficulties, create reproductive hazards and damage the bodily defences such as liver and kidneys.

Agricultural workers are commonly at risk from neurotoxic pesticides. A major study for the US Office of Technology concludes, 'All indications are that neurotoxins are a much bigger problem than originally realized.'[16] It should be no surprise that pesticides are likely to injure the biology of the brain and nervous system in some way – that is precisely how they do the job that they are designed for. Many pesticides were introduced before safety assessment was required, and remain untested. Workforces are often migrant, which makes epidemiological studies of health effects difficult. Agriculture is clearly an occupation, many of the hazards are identical to those in a factory, yet often protective legislation does not extend to agriculture. The US Occupational Safety and Health Administration lead standard, requiring employers to ensure the safety of their workers, does not apply to agricultural workers.

Research has demonstrated poorer performance in tests involving intellectual functioning, academic skills, abstraction, flexibility of thought and motor skills; memory disturbances and inability to focus attention; deficits in intelligence, reaction time and manual dexterity; and reduced perceptual speed; increased anxiety and emotional problems have also been reported.[17]

Of the more recent hazards, organophosphorus pesticides used for sheep dips have received considerable media attention. Health effects include blurred vision, slurred speech, severe headaches and memory and motor control loss. The outcome is not surprising. The chemicals are similar to those in military nerve gases first developed by the Nazis, which block cholinesterase, the enzyme needed for the brain to send nerve signals.

The hazards faced in agriculture are considerably worse in poorer countries, often because of incorrect Western assumptions about safety. Equipment used for spraying sometimes fails in countries where heat and makeshift maintenance have not been envisaged by designers. Workers often cannot read instructions, and if they can, employers encourage short-cuts. Pesticides designed for safe spraying within restricted time periods by well-nourished, healthy white males wearing protective clothing often find their way into paddy-fields where young, undernourished, unhealthy women crouch for up to 14 hours a day, immersing their genitals in pesticide-polluted water.

Because occupational health practice emanates from the richer nations, the image of 'occupation' is narrow and the concepts of regulation are often unrealistic. Informal Brazilian gold prospectors working along the River Amazon number millions, and daily inhale mercury vapour from amalgam-burning. The outcome is memory loss and other forms of 'Mad Hatter disease'. Prospectors were responsible for some 1200 tonnes of mercury entering the river by 1991, which is consumed in the form of methylmercury by those downstream who depend on the river fish for survival. The government has little power over the gold barons who control remote areas and exploit local labour.

In Java, one lead-recycling factory dumps its lead/plastic waste outside the factory gates, and villagers take this home to smelt over open fires in their back yards, extracting the last drop of the valuable metal. At first sight the arrangement seems benign. But the same factory then buys back the final product. The arrangement is simply a means to get the poor to do a form of extraction that otherwise would be commercially unviable, in a way that is very hazardous, in their own homes, outside the ambit of protective legislation. There is little comprehension in the rich nations of the levels of hazardous exposure suffered in poor countries. One study in Nicaragua found that, in a random sample of workers at the Willard battery plant, 87 per cent had blood lead levels exceeding 800 μg/litre – whereas the US federal safe level is now 100 μg/litre.[18] This was not a one-off circumstance.

Informal employment is largely ignored by the rich-nation perception. An Indian woman who earns her living by begging from cars at traffic lights might take her baby (or borrow someone else's) because this engenders sympathy. Both baby and adult will consequently suffer high levels of lead poisoning. They may then return to a home that is probably adjacent to a road, where kerosene lamps and stoves are constantly in use for domestic and informal labour, perhaps where other family members are recycling lead batteries, and with a host of other domestic threats. None of these activities is envisaged by rich-nation conceptualizations of occupational health, and their combined effect is never accounted for when 'safe' levels of exposure are fixed. WHO now promotes the idea of 'work-related' rather than 'occupational' hazards, which is far more appropriate for most of the world's population.

## Children working
In rich and poor countries alike, child labour is usually a forgotten aspect of the occupational health debate. One review terms it the tip of an 'epidemiological iceberg'.[19] If it is addressed at all, the conclusion is usually along the lines that the bodies and brains of children are particularly susceptible to toxic insults and therefore children are particularly vulnerable. But the opposite is also a possibility. There is evidence that, in specific circumstances, the young brain is less susceptible because of its plasticity and ability to construct by-passes to minor organic damage. The general health of children in impoverished settings is quite probably better than that of older people because they have had less opportunity to catch the major debilitating illnesses that increase susceptibility to toxins. Cumulative toxic effects are less likely in children. The reality is that, except in relation to a few specific hazards such as lead, the vulnerability of children (as distinct from the foetus or infant) is not known.

The 'most-vulnerable' generalization is dangerous because it can distract from other vulnerabilities in a community, and from *specific* vulnerabilities among children. Some computer models of the effects of global environmental change in the USA factor-in all under-18s as 'vulnerable'. This is a nonsense – the age group will embrace many of the fittest, healthiest, least-vulnerable members of a community. The child vulnerability debate clearly needs more refinement. Does the 'child' qualifier increase understandings of occupational health, and if so specifically how?

The main reason for the lack of concern for children is, yet again, the Western conceptualization of work which underpins research and regulation throughout the world. The safety standards for pesticides in the USA, produced by the Environmental Protection Agency (EPA) and the Occupational Safety and Health Administration (OSHA), are based only on adult exposure, for example. This ignores the reality of children working as employees or family members on farms or in market gardens.

Paradoxically, one of the reasons children become at risk in formal work settings is because of legislation that is meant to protect them. Where there are laws prohibiting or strictly regulating child labour, legal logic dictates that there cannot be specific occupational health regulations relating to children. There may be thousands of children working with toxic chemicals in the factories of a particular country, but because it is unlawful for them to do so, then they do not exist for the purposes of occupational safety legislation.

The flower industry is fast becoming one of the major threats. In Colombia children provide cheap labour for the growers, and the exposure to pesticides is extreme. Pesticide use in relation to flower production is not regulated in the same way as for food production and, as the growers are considered within the ambit of agriculture rather than industry, occupational health laws that might regulate exposure of workers producing the pesticides under controlled conditions do not apply to the children using the same chemicals in uncontrolled settings. Children are rarely protected by trade unions and if they show signs of becoming ill they are sacked before the point at which the growers are obviously accountable for health problems. Some of the pesticides used are banned in the UK and USA, yet these countries are the main importers of the flowers produced by their use.

The other work environment of children, which is rarely considered as such, is school. The classroom evades the concern of the urban environmentalist because it is considered neither home nor workplace. Throughout the world the decaying paintwork of old school buildings produces a daily threat from lead dust. It is well established that, although noise from internal classroom sources does not impair learning, noise from external sources such as traffic and trains can have a marked effect.[20] Even in wealthy nations schools are commonly sited near to main roads – where lead, particulate and noise levels are high – or adjacent to industrial areas, because such land is cheap. The infamous public poisoning by Hooker Chemical Company at Love Canal first came to light because a school baseball pitch sank into a toxic mire. The site had been bought by the Niagara Falls school board in 1953 for $1. No one thought to consider why the land was such a bargain.

As the whole purpose of the school is intellectual development, it is remarkable that planners and regulators rarely, if ever, match the school environment to the purpose of schooling by avoiding environmental threats that may diminish intellectual development. Why are the drinking-water fountains in a fifth of American schools examined still 'seriously contaminated' with lead?[21] When writing *The Lead Scandal*, Des Wilson documented the situation in the UK:

> Four primary schools are so polluted by lead and other metals that they are causing the Inner London Education Authority 'extreme concern' . . . The readings at these schools ranged from 120 ppm [parts per million] up to a staggering 26,500 ppm . . . In late 1982, sampling of lead dust in school

> *playgrounds in Hammersmith and Fulham produced further disturbing results. Of twelve schools surveyed only one had dust lead levels below the GLC guide-line of 500 ppm . . . [One] school had a range of findings from 1,550 to a terrifying 85,550.*[22]

It is hoped that these problems have now been addressed, but they probably indicate current circumstances in poorer countries.

In 1976 there was evidence that replacing cool-white fluorescent lights in classrooms with full-spectrum fluorescent tubes, which were also shielded to prevent low-frequency electromagnetic radiation, decreased hyperactive behaviour and appeared to relate to increased accomplishment. Yet cool-white tubes remain in use. The level of hazard has not been established unambiguously, but if there is a choice between one light fitting or the other, which does not have major economic implications, then why not opt for the one that appears more in accord with the purpose of a school? Since 1948 it has been argued that electromagnetic radiation is related to memory change, nervous exhaustion, headaches and subnormal EEG activity, yet never is this considered when schools are built near to electric power cables or other sources.[23]

Children's informal work settings present a range of threats which are never considered as occupational hazards. Cape Town's young newspaper sellers have blood lead levels three times greater than the official safe level. Trade unions and factory inspectors do not pay much attention to the young rag-pickers in India who dismantle and recycle the lead from car batteries or scavenge on rubbish tips where highly hazardous chemicals are dumped.

But not all street children fare badly. In many circumstances street children suffer nutritional deficiencies. But careful research in one setting found that the children on the street were better fed than their siblings who stayed at home.[24] Linda Richter concludes of South African street children

> *the longer the children spent on the streets, the worse their prognosis for educational rehabilitation. Not only did they progressively lose the basic educational skills they might have picked up in a few years of schooling, but they began to acquire handicaps. The longer the boys had spent on the streets, the more likely it was that they would show indications of cognitive and perceptual dysfunction.*[25]

But in another study the same author finds, of one-third of the group, that 'Their intellectual performance and problem-solving capacities are way above what one would predict from even better backgrounds.'[26]

Louis Aptekar comments of such findings:

> *Given the poor and impoverished beginnings why did the children seem so intelligent? It may be that street life rather than taking away from cognitive growth, actually adds to it. There are many daily activities that street children perform which are associated with improving cognitive skills, and in fact are often used in classrooms for such purposes.*[27]

Some forms of child work may be more stimulating than a poor school, although there could be a simpler explanation: that surviving street life at any level demands considerable intellectual ability, and so the population is self-selecting. But the main message from these contradictions is not complicated. Adverse conditions can, but *do not intrinsically*, threaten intellectual development of children in difficult circumstances.

## Notes

1. Y. Hennequin *et al.*, 'In-utero carbon monoxide poisoning and multiple foetal abnormalities', *The Lancet* (1993), **341**, 240.

2. *Utustan Konsumer* (1991), mid-March, p. 5.

3. M. Moore, P. Meredith and A. Goldberg, 'A retrospective analysis of blood-lead in mentally retarded children', *The Lancet* (1977), **107**, 14–25.

4. G.C. Anderson, 'Lead poisoning may last for life', *The Times*, 26 January 1996, p. 6.

5. EPA, *Preliminary Results: The Aging Solder Study* (Office of Drinking Water: Washington, DC, 1992).

6. Maureen Paul, 'Common household exposures', in Maureen Paul (ed.), *Occupational and Reproductive Hazards: A Guide for Clinicians* (Williams & Wilkins: Baltimore, DC, 1993), p. 367.

7. Andrew Hobbs, 'TV and hi-fi noise blamed for child speech problems', *Observer*, 18 July 1993, p. 3.

8. Vincent Kiernan, 'Noise pollution robs kids of language skills', *New Scientist*, 10 May 1997, p. 5.

9. DFAIT, *Global Agenda* (1996), **4**(1), 6.

10. Eric Chivian *et al.*, *Critical Condition: Human Health and the Environment* (MIT Press: Cambridge, MA, 1993), p. 62.

11. F.M. Paul, 'The problems of mental subnormality in a developing country', in Peter Mittler (ed.), *Frontiers of Knowledge in Mental Retardation*, Vol. II (International Association for the Scientific Study of Mental Deficiency: New York,1995), p. 44.

12. M. Herndez-Avila *et al.*, 'Lead-glazed ceramics as major determinants of blood lead levels in Mexican women', *Environmental Health Perspectives* (1991), **94**, 117–20.

13. Françoise Barten, *Environmental Lead Exposure of Children in Managua, Nicaragua: An Urban Health Problem* (CIP-Gegevens Koninklijke Bibliotheek: The Hague, 1992).

14. Maureen Paul (ed.), *Occupational and Reproductive Hazards: A Guide for Clinicians* (Williams & Wilkins: Baltimore, 1993).

15. D. Mergler *et al.*, 'Nervous system dysfunction among workers with long term exposure to manganese', *Environmental Research* (1994), **64**, 151–80.

16. Ellen Widess, *Neurotoxic Pesticides and the Farmworker* (OTA contract no. J3–4355.0) (Office of Technology Assessment: Washington, DC, 1988).

17. *Ibid*.

18. Barten, *op. cit*. (n. 13), p. 2

19. E.D. Richter and J. Jacobs, 'Work injuries and exposures in children and young adults: review and recommendations for action', *American Journal of Industrial Medicine* (1985), **19**, 750.

20. Sherry Ahrentzen *et al.*, 'School environments and stress', in Gary W. Williams (ed.), *Environmental Stress* (Cambridge University Press: Cambridge, 1982), p. 233.

21. G.C. Anderson, 'Lead poisoning may last for life', *The Times*, 26 January 1990.

22. Des Wilson, *The Lead Scandal: The Fight to Save Children from Damage by Lead in Petrol* (Heinemann: London, 1983).

23. Lewis W. Mayron, 'Ecological factors in learning disabilities', *Journal of Learning Disabilities* (1978), **11**(8), 499.

24. L. Aptekar, *Street Children of Cali* (Duke University Press: Durham, NC, 1988).

25. L. Richter, *Street Children: The Nature and Scope of the Problem in South Africa* (Institute for Behavioural Sciences, University of South Africa: Pretoria, 1988), p. 11.

26. L. Richter, *A Psychological Study of 'Street Children' in Johannesburg* (Institute for Behavioural Sciences, University of South Africa: Pretoria, 1988), p. 78.

27. Aptekar, *op. cit*. (n. 24).

# CHAPTER 6

# Unbounded Threats: Pollution and Disaster

The distinction between 'bounded' and 'unbounded' environments structures government reports, research, legislation and our daily perception of environmental threats. But if the divide is cloudy, particularly in poorer countries, does it have *any* analytical utility beyond convenience? If it does, the distinction should reflect the degree of power and control that individuals can exert over certain spaces, not a stereotyped view deriving from the labels we happen to give those spaces. The use of a lamp with leaded kerosene by a wealthy family in a New York loft apartment is 'bounded' in terms of their control over that hazard. But the same circumstance is very different in the Bombay slum home, where there is little control over the need to use kerosene, knowledge about the hazard is not available in a comprehensible form to enable effective decision-making and it constitutes just one of many unavoidable sources of lead leading to cumulative exposure.

From this line of thought, one aspect marks out the unbounded threats, making them worthy of a distinct approach. The degree to which political pressures attempt to construct public understandings in the unbounded sphere is quite different, because the potential cost is massive if populations become sufficiently empowered to recognize and challenge the adverse effects they suffer. The politics of research therefore becomes a central issue.

## Industry
The link between irresponsible industries and health-threatening pollution has become part of twentieth-century folklore, and needs little introduction. But, in relation to EMID, there is a danger of overlooking half of the picture. It is not just that pollutants create the *presence*-EMID threats by acting as direct neurotoxins. Because they also poison land, air and water, which creates shortages or decline in the quality of food, these pollutants are also a significant if invisible cause of *absence*-EMID, especially in poorer countries.

## Industrial disasters

Food contamination has been the easiest route through which to track the effects of industrial 'disasters'. In Taiwan in 1979, about 2000 people were poisoned by cooking oil contaminated by polychlorinated biphenyls (PCBs) and dibenzofurans. These chemicals persist in human tissue and children born to exposed mothers well after the event were affected through transplacental exposure and breast milk. They suffered a permanent five-point IQ decline, attention deficits, developmental delay, behavioural problems and a range of other adverse effects.[1] A similar circumstance was documented in Japan in 1968, which became known as *yusho* or 'oil disease'. Later studies of PCB exposure in the USA showed that mothers living around the polluted Great Lakes who eat fish from the lakes have babies with lower birth weight, smaller head size, cognitive and memory problems, and other neurological impairment. The difficulty is to isolate exactly which chemicals cause the problem.[2]

The other significant vector for poisoning is the water supply. In 1988 in Cornwall in the UK, 20 tonnes of concentrated aluminium sulphate were discharged into a treated water reservoir, causing major contamination. The official government report minimizes possible effects on the brain,[3] although a substantial out-of-court settlement was made to a few people who claimed that they had suffered adverse neurological effects. The report notes the possible link between aluminium exposure and Alzheimer's disease, acknowledging that 'it may, conceivably, accelerate the development of this disorder'. It concludes: 'there is some circumstantial evidence which suggests that exposure to aluminium over a prolonged period may contribute to age-related decline in cognitive function . . . [But we] do not consider it likely that the relatively brief increased exposure to aluminium which occurred . . . would have harmful consequences.' Although intended to deny liability, the statement embodies a tacit admission that, if the poisoning contributed to cumulative dose, there could well be an adverse effect on the brain.

These cases were well researched because they were of specific interest to the scientific community, and causation was straightforward. The Taiwan poisoning, for instance, was one of the first clear examples of an inter-generational effect from chemical exposure. More importantly perhaps, there were no strong power groups wishing to cover up what had happened.

The dumping of mercury into Minamata Bay, Japan, by Chisso and Sowa Denko in the 1950s, was probably the first example of an industrial disaster that clearly affected the human brain, and the incentive to avoid assessing the effects was strong. The problem was not acknowledged or researched for many years and remediation and compensation took decades to achieve. Fishing communities and others eating contaminated fish, numbering thousands, suffered severe intellectual disabilities, cerebral palsy, sensory impairments and speech loss, and other injuries to the central nervous system. The poison was also transmitted through breast milk. The first signs were dead fish, crazy cats and an unknown health problem among fishing communities. Initially no attempt was made to control the pollution or mitigate its effects because the polluters claimed that the inability of 1950s science to prove causal links meant that there were no links.

A more recent instance of the inability of scientific knowledge to identify impacts on the brain at the time of a disaster followed an explosion at the Hoechst Celanese chemical plant in Pampa, Texas, in 1987. The Federal Centers for Disease Control reported that the number of Down's syndrome births in Pampa was 'significantly more than expected'. The 1980s figures range from 347 to 484 Down's births each year – in a five-year period no more than two such births would normally be expected in the population. This coincided with findings from Canada that the genetic material in the sperm and egg could be disrupted before and just after conception, producing changes similar to those causing Down's syndrome. Whatever the exact cause of these Down's syndrome births in Pampa, it seems reasonable to conclude that it is not natural, and there seem few alternative explanations apart from environmental toxins.[4]

Often the severity of immediate injuries surrounding industrial disasters leads to a focus on the obvious visible problems, and longer-term effects on the brain are sidelined. Only in 1994 did the International Medical Commission on Bhopal recommend that studies of the effects of the Union Carbide poisoning should be broadened to include neurotoxicity, as existing work has been 'inadequate or extremely superficial'.[5] Tests by the Commission detecting memory loss and cognitive dysfunctions affirmed that there had been injury to the central nervous system, which had been mistaken as having a psychological cause. It is now established that 68 per cent of exposed school-going children suffered intellectual impairment, which omits the impact on those not attending school. Iatrogenic effects also contribute to the overall picture. Many of the drugs given to the Union Carbide victims were hazardous, some probably neurotoxic.

The delay between a disaster and recognition that the human intellect may be at risk is not just a poor-nation problem. At Times Beach, Missouri, in 1971, 2000 gallons of 'waste oil' were sprayed on soil at a horse arena by a contractor called Russell Bliss. Immediately, animals died and children became ill. It took three years for the government to find the cause, dioxin. The oil had been deliberately mixed with an ingredient like that used to make the herbicide Agent Orange. Eventually local people were evacuated, and Times Beach became a ghost town guarded by state troopers.

Immediate prenatal effects included hydrocephalus, and 'hyperactive children with an array of learning disabilities are common'. But it was only after longer-term study, in 1994, that Dr David Cantor, Director of Neuropsychology at the Scottish Rite Children's Medical Center, Atlanta, could conclude:

> *At first these children showed only slight signs of difficulties when dealing with elementary learning. But as they got older they experienced extreme difficulty in getting to grips with more complicated problems, problems the average child solves quite easily . . . It was obvious from this research that none of the children exposed to dioxin would ever reach their full potential as far as intelligence is concerned.*[6]

Another small-scale study of seven children found impaired attention, emotion and motivation, and that the girls suffered most. This suggests that the hormone-disrupting function of dioxin impacts in a particular way in females[7] (see Appendix).

Dioxin toxicity is very complex, which has permitted industrialists to evade responsibility for decades. In 1994, the EPA revised its view of safe levels, concluding that even at very low doses it interferes with cell development. Dioxins contaminate breast milk and cross the placenta, and some scientists now conclude that there is no 'safe level' of exposure. That dioxin is related to Agent Orange perhaps creates a disincentive within the US research community to produce firm findings about its toxicity. If the long-term threat to health is clearly established, not only might the US war veterans renew their efforts for compensation, but the Vietnamese might also demand compensation and so the broader issues of US defence policy would once again become open to question from a very emotive perspective.

## Industrial pollution

Why some happenings are labelled 'disasters' and others 'pollution' defies analysis in terms of outcome. If there is a difference, it is that pollution stems from business-as-usual operations which the public do not immediately view with surprise. Dioxins have been associated with headline disasters, but they also pervade the environment in common substances such as PVC and through processes such as paper manufacture, and are released in significant amounts through building renovations and fires. The incineration of waste accounts for 95 per cent of exposure in the USA. Major food poisonings cause national panic, but low-level daily exposures excite little interest. A US study of leading-brand baby foods found residues of eight neurotoxins and five hormone-disrupting pesticides.[8] The main consequence of the pollution label is that redress is even less likely than when the disaster label is applied.

Brazil's biggest industrial complex is located in Cubatão, near São Paulo. At one time over 20 tonnes of pollutants were emitted each day. Residents in a *favela* on the edge of the city were most at risk. One of the most common birth impairments was anencephaly – the brain is partially or completely missing – which is easily recognized because of the shape of the skull. The normal incidence is one case per 5000 births. In Cubatão, in 1982, it was one per 300; in 1981 one per 200. The official explanation was that malnutrition, alcohol and smoking were the cause. And as is so often the case, the whistle-blowers were silenced or discredited. Romeu Magalheas, a local hospital doctor, was sacked when he stated that he intended to make the facts more widely known.[9]

Not all hazards come from heavy industry. Those living near dry-cleaning shops are likely to suffer from low-level exposure to tetrachloroethylene (TCE). German researchers found that vigilance, simple reaction time and visual memory were significantly affected 'despite the low exposure levels . . . if the exposure lasts for several years'. They conclude, 'the results justify any effort to limit exposure to TCE of people living in the vicinity of dry cleaning facilities'.[10]

But local problems such as this appear insignificant in the light of pollution the other side of the former Berlin Wall, which again raises the question about what gets researched where and why. In Copsa Mica, Romania, the IMMN factory smelts lead, cadmium, zinc and copper. Everything within 20 miles is blackened. Reports concluded that it has 'poisoned the inhabitants with lead and cadmium, and damaged children's intelligence'. Blood lead levels in children are twice permitted levels, and children are scoring 'markedly worse than usual' results in IQ tests.[11] Elsewhere in the former Soviet bloc the picture is similar. At polluted Magnitogorsk, in Russia, it is reported that birth defects have doubled since 1980. Space in homes for mentally retarded youngsters is 'at a premium' and children are simply warehoused in wards with barely room to walk between the beds.[12] But these are only anecdotal reports – there are no formal studies.

The spotlight on the former communist countries is to some extent a continuation of Cold War propaganda, which can also conveniently distract from pollution problems in the non-communist states. In 1994 a report about the North American Great Lakes, by an International Joint Commission, linked increased pollution to reproductive health problems and developmental problems in children. The commission made the obvious recommendations but they were not new. They reflected environmental regulations that had been in place for 22 years.

Pollution should be controlled by environmental risk assessment – a Western concept that fails to acknowledge cultural dynamics. In 1994 the Ugba River in Nigeria was polluted by industrial waste from Benin City, which turned the water red. As a result of people in Ulemon Village drinking the water for two years, there were numerous premature births and babies born with impairments. The reason that village people drank the water was not just ignorance of the risk, but that they thought that its sudden change in colour was a message from the gods. Capitalist hazards are minimized, communist legacies hyped, but non-Western cultural dynamics have yet to enter the frame. And this applies to most of the world's population.

## Agriculture

Making a distinction between industry and agriculture is rapidly becoming meaningless. But it does embody one important characteristic – the direct threat to the food supply. Not least, we now know that air pollution is reducing crop yields around cities in Asia.[13]

In Iraq in 1971–2 farmers mistakenly used a seed grain treated with a methylmercury fungicide to make bread, leading to the hospitalization of 6530 people. Some of the children who suffered severe poisoning had permanent physical and mental disabilities. Mild cognitive dysfunction was common.[14] In similar previous incidents, farmers thought that washing the grain would remove the mercury. In the 1971 case some had tested the grain by feeding it to farm animals, and concluded that the absence of any adverse effect meant that it was safe for human consumption.

A more recent case in Hungary demonstrates the threat from new and untested substances, and, like the Iraq case, the important factors ignored by formal risk assessment: human failing and human necessity. In 1988–90 Trichlorfon, an organophosphorus insecticide, was introduced to eradicate parasites in fish farms in an area around Rinya. Fish died, but local people were not told about the possible hazard. Although fishing was officially prohibited, the impoverished villagers caught fish by hand and ate them. In one village, of 15 births by mothers who had eaten the fish, 11 had congenital abnormalities, and four of these had Down's syndrome.[15] After people had stopped eating the fish, ten later births were without clinical problems. The insecticide had been used undiluted, which was not in accord with instructions.

In the light of these cases it is astounding to find the Scottish Environmental Protection Agency, in 1996, sanctioning the use of ivermectin, a neurotoxin, to eradicate sea lice in salmon farmed off south Skye. John Duffins, Director of the Edinburgh Centre for Toxicology, warned that, even without human error, the toxin might be a reproductive hazard. It also accumulates in human body fats, and could then be released in later life when stored fat is used to fight the diseases of old age.[16]

While poisonings make the most dramatic headlines, history is likely eventually to put the Green Revolution at the top of the list of agricultural threats to intellectual resources. To solve world food shortages in the 1950s, the Green Revolution introduced high-yield rice, wheat and maize varieties. But these varieties are low in minerals and vitamins, and the Revolution also displaced traditional sources of micro-nutrients – local fruits, vegetables and legumes. In 1992 a UN report formally recorded concern. One result is iron deficiency, which, in recent years, is the only nutritional problem to have worsened worldwide. Further long-term impacts will come from degraded land, fertilizer and pesticide residues and water shortages – the foreseeable but unforeseen by-products of the Green Revolution.

The paradox then is that even as the food supply in some countries has increased, so has the number of people suffering incapacitating vitamin and mineral deficiencies . . . [The] deficiencies strike at one of the major forces that drive progress – intellectual resources. Improving primary school education is one of the most efficient ways to fuel a country's advancement, but the opportunity can be wasted on children who are lacking certain key vitamins and minerals because they may simply be incapable of learning.[17]

Agricultural science may, of course, help to prevent EMID. In highly polluted regions of Poland, special types of crops that do not take up heavy metals from the soil as readily as standard varieties are being grown. But optimism may be false. These varieties of crops are likely not to take up other minerals from the soil, and this then creates the *absence*-EMID micro-nutrient deficiencies. Those affected are then more likely to ingest heavy metals from other sources, so the overall threat to intellectual resources could be back to square one.

## Nuclear power generation
Nuclear power exemplifies the cover-up dynamics of disaster and pollution politics, not least because the industry is, or was, primarily conceived for military purposes. Even a simple fundraising advert from Greenpeace can meet immediate resistance (see Chapter 1). Unfortunately, high-profile debates such as these have distracted from the growing, but rarely noticed, incremental evidence of the threats posed to the human brain by nuclear power. No longer can the nuclear industry claim that its activities are

unrelated to intellectual decline. Following the radiation release at Three Mile Island, a damages payment of $1 million was made to a boy born with Down's syndrome nine months later.

In 1957, radioactive fallout from an unplanned release at the ill-fated British power station, Windscale, was known to have reached Ireland at a time of heavy rainfall over the town of Dundalk. An increased incidence of Down's syndrome along the east coast of Ireland, peaking in 1974, was noted, and a link was made with mothers attending the same school in Dundalk. Six out of 26 babies were born with the syndrome, which was 'far too high to be the result of chance alone' – the usual rate was one in 600. The conclusion was that exposure to radiation, perhaps combined with an influenza-like infection, had precipitated the condition.[18]

A study by Dr John Bound and co-workers notes that ground contamination from the Windscale release coincided with increased fallout from weapons testing, which he linked to increased prevalence of Down's syndrome in Lancashire.[19] That older women were more at risk (even after controlling for the age factor) is explained by additive effects of exposure to low doses. It is commonly argued that exposure from nuclear power *or* weapons testing is too small to have any effect. The Bound study suggests that even small exposures might be significant, if cumulative.

There is little doubt that the Soviet nuclear power disaster at Chernobyl has had similar effects in that region, and radiation does not stop at national boundaries. A study of an increase in babies born with Down's syndrome in Germany, nine months after the explosion, concluded unambiguously 'that the increased prevalence of trisomy 21 [Down's syndrome] in West Berlin in January 1987 was causally related to a short period of exposure to ionizing radiation as a result of the Chernobyl reactor accident'.[20] There was a cluster of 12 cases in a population in which two or three might be expected. A follow-up study by the Human Genetics Institute of (the then) West Berlin found that of 17 babies born with Down's syndrome, 15 were from the most heavily contaminated region in the south.[21] A similar increase in the rate of Down's syndrome was also observed for infants born in 1987 in the Lothian region of Scotland, in Sweden and in Denmark.[22]

The significance of these studies is less in what they reveal and more in what they remind of. If such outcomes are detectable hundreds of miles from the disaster, what happened near Chernobyl? We do not know because Soviet secrecy, cash shortages, political pressures and logistical problems prevented proper assessment. The estimate that 15 children were born mentally retarded, by the US Nuclear Regulatory Commission, was almost certainly too low. The figure of 100 is more probable.[23]

Headline disasters are not the only cause for concern. In 1991 a federal study in Canada found an extremely high incidence of Down's syndrome in two communities near the Pickering nuclear power station, Ontario: 86 per cent higher than the provincial average in Pickering and 46 per cent above in Ajax; a total of 38 children with Down's syndrome. The report concluded that further investigation 'would be prudent', and the Canadian Atomic Energy Control Board (AECB) admitted that the plant regularly released small amounts of tritium, causing 'very small doses to the population in the vicinity' of reactors.

A subsequent study by the Canadian AECB dismissed the original findings on the basis that the Down's syndrome births did not fit a pattern of high releases of tritium.[24] But as John Bound concludes, from his UK study of fall-out from weapons testing (above), the genetic injury may arise because of a *cumulative* dose suffered by the mother. If this is so, it is immaterial whether or not the Down's syndrome births fit a pattern of high or low releases. The AECB then recommended 'further research' to examine 'other possible contributing factors such as medical x-ray exposures and the occupations of both parents'. The use of the words 'other' and 'contributing' are curious, because this could amount to an admission that the tritium was at least in part responsible for the genetic damage. Pickering releases may have been the final-straw factor, and courts could award damages on this basis.

In the research world, what does *not* happen is sometimes more telling than what does. From China there appears to be only one study making a link between high levels of background radiation and Down's syndrome, in Yangjiang, and the radiation source is natural.[25] From India there seems also to be only one location worthy of mainstream research in relation to radiation EMID. This too relates to a natural occurrence, in Kerala.[26] Bearing in mind the extent of the military and civil nuclear programmes in China and India, it would be remarkable if natural occurrences provided the only settings worth researching. (Gadelar's work, detailed later, is an exception, but this has not penetrated the mainstream literature.) And these two areas of study represent the sum of human knowledge concerning radiation EMID in relation to over one-third of the world's population.

While most research has focused on atmospheric radiation, the threat posed from careless disposal of waste might be far greater. In 1994, Russian scientists revealed that billions of gallons of nuclear waste had been pumped below ground into shale and clay at sites at Dimitrovgrad near the Volga River, Tomsk near the Ob River and Krasnoyarsk on the Yenisei, and that waste had spread a great distance. From Tibet there are press reports of a significant increase in birth impairments around dumps for Chinese nuclear waste.[27]

Similarly, to concentrate on radiation may be to miss the broader threats posed by nuclear power. The building and maintenance of such stations calls for the production and use of massive amounts of toxic substances, including mercury and lead for shielding. Lead powder is used in the rubber sheeting used to make protective clothing, the manufacture and disposal of which significantly increases the hazard posed by lead.

In Rawatbhata, Rajasthan, Dr Sanghamitra Gadekar carried out an unofficial study of 3000 villagers who live around the Rajasthan Atomic Power Station. She found extreme levels of disability, including Down's syndrome and 'a new generation with an increased number of deformed babies without fingers, jointed toes, missing genital organs and abnormal sized heads'.[28] The responsible agencies argue that it cannot be proven that these disabilities are caused by radiation, because they may be the result of the poverty, poor nutrition and poor health of the villagers. As an academic exercise, let us for a moment accept the official argument – and then ask what is the cause of the poverty, nutrition and health problems. It is only necessary to look at the landscape around the power station to see the environmental degradation it has caused. Toxic tips abound, the streams froth with toxins and the soil is nearly useless. In Rawatbhata, even if radiation has not caused disability, the nuclear power station almost certainly has.

It is not just the poorer countries that suffer this problem. In 1993 British Nuclear Fuels Ltd admitted that non-radioactive toxic chemicals had leaked into the River Calder from the Sellafield (formerly Windscale) reprocessing plant. The story received little media attention because the stereotype is that radiation is the only threat associated with nuclear power. Perhaps the main difference in the poorer nations is that we can see the effects of such toxic waste. Better waste management in the richer nations does not mean no effect. Research about the environmental consequences of nuclear power needs to broaden its focus beyond the high-profile, scientifically sexy concern with radiation.

## Transnational exploitation
For families such as those which exist by scavenging on the waste tip in Oruro, Bolivia, the disaster/pollution, bounded/unbounded distinctions are meaningless. Even the boundaries of nations failed to protect them. The 500 tonnes of toxic slag – containing lead, arsenic, chromium and other heavy metals – that constitutes their workplace, meeting-place, home and children's playground was never labelled a disaster because the slag originated from a tin smelter in Humberside, UK. The slag should have been reprocessed, but was instead dumped and forgotten.

Such deceit seems common. In 1992, US companies exported 3000 tonnes of fertilizer to Bangladesh, with assistance from the Asian Development Bank. It contained 1000 tonnes of toxic waste, including heavy metals, which was secretly mixed in before export. If intent was deliberately to poison a nation's children, there could be few better ways. According to a worker at the Produquimica chemical plant in the Mata Atlantica rainforest, Brazil, 'People are being poisoned by mercury, lead, becoming blind, mad.' The source is again the UK. To evade import restrictions, a toxic cocktail of lead, mercury, cadmium, arsenic and cobalt was described as 'micronutrients for fertilizer production'.

Of all the disasters exported to the poor nations, car batteries are probably the most devastating. Children from the Philippines, Indonesia, Taiwan, Thailand, Mexico, Brazil and China are recipients.[29] In Malaysia, battery workers at foreign-managed plants have lead levels three times the US health limits. If workers and children survive the lead, when PVC casings are burned this creates dioxin; other processes produce cadmium. The list of countries on the receiving end of the disaster export trade is not so dissimilar from the list of countries receiving bilateral aid for building schools. The intellectual resources of recipient countries might have been better served if the donor countries had kept their cash – and kept their toxic waste.

The work of Greenpeace and others in the early 1990s told the world of toxic exports such as these, which were clearly against the spirit of international agreements but not directly outlawed because companies termed the trade 'recycling', not export. Eventual agreement within the Basel Convention in 1994 may have blocked this loophole, but while congratulating itself on agreeing that toxic exports had been wrong, the international community took no measures to compensate victims or mitigate damage already done. If UK doctors cause a British child to suffer brain injury at birth, they are considered culpable and financial compensation reflects the need for special support throughout the child's lifetime. If UK company directors cause brain damage to hundreds of children in other countries, through exporting tonnes of toxic waste, it seems that they can forget all about it because their government has signed an international convention.

The export of toxic waste is paralleled by the export of toxic factories. One of the outcomes of environmental and workplace legislation in the USA has been that dirty industries have relocated to Mexico, to the infamous *maquiladoras* factories which employ half a million Mexicans at around $4 to $10 per day. A disturbing increase in developmental disability has been reported by the Matamoros School for Special Education. One hundred and ten affected children, known as the 'Malory children', were born to 76 mothers who worked in a factory of that name, where solvents containing lead were manufactured in unsafe conditions. In Matamoros, 53 anencephalic (brainless) children were born within 1990–2. This is mirrored on the US side of the border, in Brownsville, Texas, where there were 30 cases – three were born within 36 hours at one health centre. The incidence is three to four times the US average. Mothers in Brownsville sued the Mexican factories for disabilities and death caused, they claim, by the toxic cocktail of chemicals blown across the border. This is an ironic twist when it is remembered that the root cause of the problem is exploitation from the US side.

> . . . suddenly all the environmental knowledge accumulated over a generation is denied. When industrialists along the border are challenged about the effects of their pollution, the arguments have to begin from zero. Medical staff have to prove that pesticides ingested could be harmful; that lead can cause brain damage; that children wading barefoot in toxic waste might be at risk. (Peter Lennon, writing about the *maquiladoras* industries on the USA–Mexico border[30])

## Commercial abuse of power

Beyond direct transnational exploitation, many of the threats posed by commercial abuse of power are less tangible than disasters or pollution. Smoking by mothers affects the birth weight of their babies, and low birth weight is linked to developmental problems. When tobacco companies aim their advertising specifically at children, or spray tobacco leaves with additional nicotine, doubling the dose intentionally to increase addiction, the consequences go well beyond increased tobacco consumption and lung disease. The aggressive advertising of junk foods with low nutritional value and additives that can affect behaviour is a similar abuse of power.

The excessive promotion of artificial milk over breast milk is a form of social manipulation that is generally taken to threaten intellectual resources. According to UNICEF, children fed with artificial milk demonstrate IQ levels on average 8.3 per cent lower than those fed naturally.[31] One reason is that artificial milk lacks long-chain polyunsaturated fatty acids, which are considered essential for optimum brain development.[32] Work from University Hospital, Groningen, suggests that bottle-fed babies are twice as likely to suffer brain dysfunction. The argument can be put more simply. Cows' milk, the basis of artificial versions, is designed to nourish offspring with a massive body and a small, unintellectual brain. Human milk is designed for the reverse case.

One study contradicting this general contention concluded that dummy use, not bottle-feeding, was a marker of a lower IQ.[33] But this was based on an assessment of the intelligence of adults aged 50 to 60, and much could have happened to change IQ in the interim. Of course, artificial milk used appropriately is a crucial part of improving the nutritional status of a nation's children. So, remembering the thread of this and the preceding chapter, the problem is not artificial milk, but what we do with it.

## Industrial discourse

The discourse of disaster and pollution could consume a book on its own. Industrial disasters are often described misleadingly as 'accidents'. The poisoning perpetrated by the Union Carbide Factory in Bhopal, for instance, stemmed from reckless disregard for safety standards -- it was not an accident. Common law, concerning assault for example, makes a distinction between 'deliberate', 'reckless' and 'accidental' acts. Only the latter is a defence. Accurate phraseology is imperative to achieve a clear public perception, because this may ultimately be reflected in a jury decision.

It is also curious how those bound up in science can forget their baseline: the natural human condition that permitted human survival for millions of years, without science or technology. When discussing existing research about the link between breastfeeding and intelligence, researchers state: 'Although these findings suggest that breastfeeding in early life may promote cognitive development, their interpretation is complicated.'[34] What do they mean by 'promote'? Breastfeeding is not an off-the-shelf brain tonic – it is the natural way in which human infants are nourished, permitting a normal, unimpeded development. The message from research about breastfeeding is that artificial substitutes may *diminish* intellectual potential from the natural norm, not that breastfeeding can promote it.

Why too do disasters come to be known by their geographical location and not by the name of the responsible entity? It is no doubt of great comfort to perpetrators that we talk of the 'Bhopal', 'Times Beach' and 'Chernobyl' disasters, rather than of the Union Carbide, Russell Bliss or nuclear industry crimes. Why has community poisoning by the Hooker Chemical and Plastics Corporation come to be known by a phrase that otherwise would be taken as the title of a B movie: Love Canal? This discourse is not so very far removed from talking of Jack the Ripper as the 'London disaster'.

## Traffic

Traffic is usually seen as posing a threat to the brain through airborne pollutants, principally lead. In the USA, arguments about the cost of not protecting children have culminated in increasingly strict controls. By contrast, in China there is no unleaded petrol and car ownership will increase by a million a year from the year 2000. In Poland less than 1 per cent of petrol is lead-free. African petrol has the highest lead content in the world – three times greater than elsewhere. In the UK, the introduction of unleaded petrol at a cheaper price than leaded, but without a mandatory phase-out, has encouraged only half of Britain's motorists to change to unleaded. Perhaps this sounds encouraging, but it is possible that any potential benefit will be reduced by the increase in car miles driven each year by those still using leaded petrol.

Politics abound. Professor Derek Bryce-Smith warned of the dangers of leaded petrol in the 1950s, and was rewarded with ridicule and professional and political marginalization in the UK. In retrospect, few find serious fault with his work. Cars *can* run without lead in petrol, at no extra cost to car manufacturers or petrol companies. The block is the lobbying power of the companies that make leaded petrol. Above all other hazards, the lead-in-petrol debate has constantly displayed how governments put profits before prophets.[35]

The leaded-petrol industry argues that petrol is one of many sources of lead, and so it cannot be singled out for blame. Campaigners traditionally respond by isolating data about petrol to counter this argument. The outcome then stands or falls on whether or not lead in petrol alone poses a threat – a line of debate that favours the leaded-petrol industry. More effective is to argue the cumulative effect of environmental lead, of which exposure to traffic emissions is an inescapable contributor. Lead pollution near a motorway might be below a supposed safe level, but an exposure to two 'safe' sources doubles the hazard, not the safety factor.

> She was three years old and lived in decaying inner city housing where she was exposed to old leaded paint and to exhaust emissions from heavy passing traffic . . . her brain was swollen – a condition known as encephalopathy, the result of severe lead poisoning. I treated her with chelating agents and she recovered. I felt triumphant . . . Then when I told the mother that her daughter couldn't go back into that home she asked me, 'Where am I going to move? Every house on the block is the same.' Confronted by those realities I began to realize that it is not enough just to give a drug. The disease is out there in the world, not just in the child. (Dr Herbert L. Needleman)[36]

The attention to lead in petrol can obscure other hazards. The manufacture and disposal of batteries is a massive problem, especially in poorer countries. Ethylene dibromide is also a neurotoxic petrol additive, yet we hear little about it. All petrol creates dioxin pollution – leaded nine times more than unleaded – which can disrupt hormones (see Appendix). At low levels of exposure carbon monoxide slows thought processes, impairs vision and causes headaches and drowsiness. It is interesting to conjecture the possible increase in productivity in city offices if this single environmental toxin were absent. We know that particulates can enter the brain,[37] but not the effect. Polish research found that babies exposed *in utero* to high levels of PM10 particles are born with smaller heads, which could impair their learning.[38]

In many countries – Kuwait, for example – road traffic accidents appear to be a far more significant cause of childhood disability than pollutants.[39] Using an innovative approach to statistics, researchers from Heidelberg conclude that every 100 cars are responsible for one handicapped person.[40] The emphasis that is usually put on chemical rather than physical causes, concerning traffic, exemplifies how Western scientific approaches can overshadow common-sense notions of causality when arguing for preventive measures. In some settings, safe pedestrian crossings or traffic calming may be as important as unleaded petrol.

Even if pollutants had no direct effect on the brain, the indirect consequences of traffic for intellectual development are significant. The debate about the degree to which traffic pollution is linked to the increase in respiratory ailments in children fluctuates daily, but there is some agreement that particulates certainly precipitate latent, or exacerbate existing, conditions. Children sitting in their classroom coughing or fighting for breath are unlikely to be giving their full attention to their lessons.

The increased physical presence of traffic has other less obvious implications. A study by the UK Policy Studies Institute notes that in 1971, 80 per cent of 7- and 8-year-olds went to school on their own; by 1993, only 9 per cent did so. The reason is that more parents take children to school in cars. The effects on children are an inability to 'develop coping skills, self-esteem, a sense of identity, the capacity to take responsibility, and to use their minds creatively'.[41]

Iatrogenicity (cures that cause ills), this time in a technical form, is a neglected aspect of the traffic debate. For example, catalytic converters may filter out some of the pollutants related to respiratory disease, but, if entering the air in a sufficient quantity, cadmium particles from the converters themselves may eventually create a hazard to the brain. The most problematic iatrogenicity conundrum concerns electric cars, which might at first appear the obvious cure for urban pollution. But a study from Carnegie-Mellon University in Pittsburgh claims that, because of the increased use of lead for batteries, electric cars will consequently release 60 times more lead per kilometre of use, relative to a comparable car burning leaded gasoline.[42] Electric cars alter, rather than remove, the lead threat associated with traffic. The stories of unregulated lead smelters and children's involvement in the battery-recycling industry remind us that the findings from Carnegie-Mellon might be an underestimation in the context of poorer nations.

Ultimately, the solution to environmental threats caused by traffic is to reduce traffic. And this is largely a social, not technical problem.

## War

War is rarely considered as a cause of intellectual disability, yet the broad environmental links are very obvious. The destruction of hospitals, water supplies, sanitation and other infrastructure has a direct toll on the health of infants and children. In Iraq, protein-, vitamin- and calorie-related malnutrition has increased by a factor of 11 since the Gulf War. Low birth weight has increased fourfold, leading to assessments that Iraq will have millions of stunted children. Other birth difficulties can also be war-related. In Sarajevo's Kosevo hospital, in 1993, 15 per cent of births were of children with impairments, which was attributed to stress, poor diet and poor pre-natal care.

The outcome of relatively minor damage to the toxic time bombs, such as chemical factories or electrical transformers which release PCBs when they catch fire, can be as destructive in the long term as the immediate effects of military action. An unpublished UN report in 1994 warned that pollution of the Danube by toxins from the Balkan conflict – dioxins, PCBs and heavy metals – could significantly increase the numbers of children born with congenital malformations. The destruction of a factory at Osijek released 100 tonnes of chemicals used to make pesticides, in undiluted form.

Specific military strategies create direct hazards. Mines are usually associated with the loss of limbs, but some are designed to shoot canisters into the air to inflict head injuries. The effects of dioxin in Agent Orange, the defoliant used in the Vietnam War, were contested by the US government for more than ten years. Although now accepting that exposure can cause certain cancers, a 1993 study by the US National Academy of Science's Institute of Medicine still ignores neurological disorders and birth impairments, although both have been demonstrated in animal experiments.

The initial reluctance of the British government to instigate research into the so-called Gulf War syndrome displayed a desire not to discover the truth when military service was seen as a cause of a host of adverse outcomes among veterans, which included memory loss and concentration problems. Birth impairments in children fathered by US veterans have ten times the normal prevalence rate, according to Ohio paediatrician Francis

Waickman. In one Mississippi unit, of 16 babies born after the war, 13 suffered. In 1994, six UK veterans sued the Ministry of Defence on behalf of babies born with impairments.

The chemical soup to which soldiers were exposed included depleted uranium dust from US anti-tank shells, organophosphate pesticides, heavy metals in the smoke from burning oil wells, perhaps chemical weapons and iatrogenic effects – the untested drugs administered to prevent the effects of chemical exposure. Whatever the truth of the Gulf War syndrome, it raises an important ethical question. While it is generally accepted that non-conscript soldiers tacitly accept any risk associated with war, can they accept a risk on behalf of their unborn children?

Protest from US Vietnam and Gulf War veterans, though certainly not unwarranted, disguises a broader question: what of the effects on those on the receiving end? There has been relatively little interest, from the scientific community, in the suffering caused to Vietnamese and Iraqi children. The use of uranium-tipped shells and bullets has left 40 tonnes of depleted uranium in the Gulf War battle zone, according to the UK Atomic Energy Agency. This will not disappear for centuries, and children use the old shell cases as toys. Even if Agent Orange had no direct neurotoxic effect, result-ant ecological damage would obviously cause malnutrition, which would significantly affect children. The USA is not cautioned by the Vietnam War. Its 1987 'War on Drugs' in Guatemala involved the spraying of marijuana and opium poppies with highly toxic defoliants, and this was undertaken with no concern about the effects on the children of the farmers.

> People are still living with the effects of Agent Orange and dioxin used during the war. We see cleft palates, heart defects, children born with no arms or legs. They're often abandoned. (Christina Noble, who runs a shelter for Vietnamese street children[43])

History may eventually conclude that, since the Second World War, the manufacture rather than the use of weapons has posed the greater threat to human life and health. On a small scale Nicaragua provides an example. From 1984, the contra-revolution increased the demand for batteries. There was a resultant growth of the battery manufacturing plants and related cottage industries in Managua, and increased adverse effects on children from haphazard lead production and use.[44]

Toxin weapons are specifically designed to target the brain and central nervous system. The use of such weapons has been rare, but the testing, manufacture, storage and disposal inevitably leads to exposure of workers and the public. In 1995, 25,000 tonnes of chemical weapons – including nerve agents, mustard gas, phosgene gas and toxic seed dressings – were discovered in the Irish Sea. Since the dumping at the end of the Second World War, there has been no monitoring of possible pollution.

The consequences of abandoning normal industrial safety practices in munitions manufacturing are most evident in the former Soviet Union. As the Cold War ended, the world learned of the health problems suffered by those who worked in the military industrial cities and of the secrecy surrounding this situation. One press report described a city called 'No. 19', near Moscow, which was for forty years engaged in making nuclear and chemical weapons. It told how a TV film showing 'a bus that was full of children with terrible deformities' was confiscated before it could be shown.[45] In the Chuvash region, where nerve gas was produced, chronic child disease is 40 per cent higher than elsewhere. Soviet weapons and their manufacturing plants were probably safer during the Cold War, because at that time they at least had an intrinsic value.

But it is misleading to think that this circumstance pertained only in the former USSR. The US Department of Defense has admitted to 18,000 toxic hot spots in 2000 of its bases. In Nevada, a secret airforce base, known as Area 51 or 'Dreamland', was not acknowledged to exist by the US military. Workers and communities are known to have been exposed to dioxins, methylethylketone, trichlorethylene and dibenzofurans. Soviet intelligence pictures of the base have appeared in British newspapers, but if the US government maintains the line that the base does not exist, no one can sue for adverse health effects.

## Nuclear weapons

It might seem self-evident that dropping an A-bomb on a community is likely to damage the brains of babies *in utero*. But it has taken the US scientific community 45 years to conclude formally that there was 'a major (and dose–response-related) increase in severe mental retardation', together with sub-clinical effects on school performance, among survivors of the US A-bombs dropped on Hiroshima and Nagasaki.[46] The decline in school performance was 'highly significant' among those exposed between 8 to 15 and 16 to 25 weeks after conception.

If the threat only concerned the *use* of nuclear weapons, there might be little more to discuss, but, as indicated above, it is the process of manufacturing and testing that has posed the most significant hazard. Some proponents of the nuclear deterrent claim that the Cold War cost no lives, yet over time nuclear weapons are likely to have killed and injured large numbers of people. It is not just that those injured are non-combatants; they are not even the enemy. They are neither perceived by the public nor accepted by governments as victims of war.

In 1969, Dr Ernest Sternglass estimated that 400,000 US infants had died because of nuclear testing.[47] Sternglass was not a natural opponent of nuclear development – he was a physicist working at Westinghouse. The US Center for Defense Information acknowledged in 1991 that communities downwind of the Nevada test site have an incidence of thyroid cancers that is eight times the norm; bone cancers twelve times. Some public exposure was not by accident. In the USA many releases of radioactivity and toxins such as mercury were 'routine' means of disposal. Some releases were deliberate experiments. In 1949 the Hanford nuclear weapons facility exposed 270,000 people to radioactivity to test fallout-sensing monitors.

> We had a lot of mental retardation. This had become very apparent early in 1956 . . . there had never been even a need for a class, and all of a sudden these children of Layne's age, here were twelve or so in one class . . . We had all these children that needed special education, who were not only slightly handicapped but severely retarded. These were extremely retarded children. It really struck us. We said, they were all born during that time, how come?
>
> . . . If we go back and see the perception of people, it wasn't like now . . . Retardation was something to hide and to keep away from people. Above all you would not admit it openly to your friends. Now we say they are Down's syndrome, and in those days they were Mongolian idiots . . . Who would want to teach in front of a class, would even want to be seen with them? . . .
>
> All of a sudden we had all these children desperately needing schooling, training. Parents were totally frustrated, really hiding things they couldn't handle . . . We were the first ones in the state of Utah to have a trainable class unit in a school. Up to that time they would get a few of them together and hide them in a building someplace where nobody could see them, where nobody could make contact with them.
>
> . . . I don't think we need to be compensated. I don't think compensation solves the problem. I don't think other citizens in another part of the country need to pay us – they weren't at fault either . . . To be in apology and acknowledgment, and to clean up the act so that they [the government] can be trusted again. I would fight like anything to get that to happen, if I knew what to do. (Sheldon and Leatrice Johnson, St George, Utah. Parents of a boy with Down's syndrome)[48]

There is now no dispute that exposure to low-level ionizing radiation can cause intellectual decline. But for decades it has been denied that background radiation from weapons testing has posed any threat. In 1994, a study linking Down's syndrome to low-dose radiation, in the UK, found that the rate of the syndrome peaked at the time of high, whole-body radiation doses from fallout from nuclear testing. In one instance the prevalence rocketed from 67 to 431 cases per 10,000 births. The researcher Dr John Bound concluded: 'It seems that the total dose you've had in your life is much more important than any individual dose. The greater susceptibility of older women suggests that these low doses may be the straw that broke the camel's back.'[49]

The argument that exposure due to nuclear testing is usually lower than background radiation from natural sources therefore becomes open to question, because it may be the additive effect of natural and human-made sources (including power stations) that triggers the genetic damage. The probability becomes more tangible in other settings. Radioactive fallout in the Ural weapons testing area is more than twice that from the Soviet nuclear power disaster at Chernobyl.[50]

Radiation exposure does not result only from testing. The mining of uranium at the Wismut complex near Leipzig, Germany, has left a legacy of toxic tips containing 718 million cubic feet of contaminated dust, which blows over an area inhabited by 1.2 million people. Cancer rates are very high, and it is reported that 'thousands are disabled because of the radiation in the area'.[51]

As with civil uses, to concentrate only on radiation can be misleading. The production of nuclear weapons involved a host of other threats. In 1977, a report from Union Carbide about its Y-12 factory at Oak Ridge, Tennessee, admitted that it had 'lost' 2.4 million pounds of mercury since 1953. The highest levels of mercury pollution ever recorded were found in an adjacent stream, much of it entering Poplar Creek. The consequences were never fully evaluated, nor people warned not to eat fish from the river, because much of the necessary information was classified.[52]

Most of our data about radiation and war come from Hiroshima and Nagasaki. But we hear little about research concerning the US weapons-testing zones, where the numbers suffering intellectual decline and other health effects seem also to be very high. Much of the Japanese research was carried out by American scientists. Why did some not stay at home, where the logistics of research could have been far easier? It is convenient for American military history that this form of time-latent war injury is something that appears to happen only to the enemy.

## Unbounded lessons

One of the victims of the Russell Bliss dioxin poisoning at Times Beach concluded, 'If we were exotic animals, the government would have protected us, but we are not an endangered species.'[53] She is only half right.

Rarity is not the key factor in denial – being human is. Even if causation is admitted, animals don't sue. And, together with military interests, this dynamic underpins the politics of the unbounded environmental threats, with which the research world is often tacitly or knowingly complicit.

In *The Politics of Mental Handicap*, Joanna Ryan makes the simple point that researchers 'tend to be more interested in investigating the extremely rare but scientifically more definable symptoms . . . rather than trying to promote social action that would reduce the commoner but less clear-cut forms of mental handicap'.[54] The pattern is very evident in relation to EMID: the emphasis on radiation rather than toxic waste from nuclear power stations, on chemical emissions from traffic rather than accidents, on chemical weapons rather than infrastructure damage from war, on micro-nutrient deficiencies rather than general poverty. This is not to conclude that we should not take note of all aspects – and comprehend the synergistic and cumulative effects – but the more mundane problems should not be pushed aside in the wake of scientific fashion. The result otherwise is to collude with the interests of the polluters – the scientifically interesting problems will nearly always be on a smaller scale.

Research reports, especially in relation to radiation, give the impression of only one EMID outcome – Down's syndrome – and the numbers of children affected will always appear minimal. But this is misleading. The main reason that Down's syndrome features prominently is that it is one of the few unambiguous manifestations of intellectual disability. Clinical diagnosis is simple. Initial screening can rely on inquiries within a general community because people with Down's syndrome have distinctive facial features, which is especially useful in poorer countries where medical records may be inadequate. In the Kerala study mentioned above, the authors state quite clearly, 'Only gross abnormalities evident on clinical examination were recorded.'

The managers of a hazardous industrial endeavour, such as a nuclear power station, might confidently commission research about Down's syndrome knowing that, because this can occur naturally, causation is difficult to establish, and even if a link is conclusive the numbers who suffer will probably seem too small to precipitate widespread public concern. A painstaking but clinically uninteresting study of school achievement might reveal a much bigger outcome.

Similarly, informal reports often concern anencephaly (the complete or partial absence of a brain), which is obvious from a misshaped head and makes effective press photos. Although sad, anencephaly does not directly pose a significant threat to intellectual resources of a community because such children usually die quickly. Again, the numbers affected will appear small, and can appear unimportant when compared by politicians or industrialists against statistics concerning, say, brain injury from traffic accidents.

The fuller picture comes from remembering the unclear divide between clinical and sub-clinical outcomes, such as the Hiroshima evidence. Clinical mental handicap is so often just the tip of a sub-clinical iceberg. In research findings, Down's syndrome and other conspicuous outcomes are just indicators, not definitive conclusions about the prevalence of EMID. To think otherwise not only colludes with the politics of the perpetrator, but clouds the answer to the main question of *Terminus Brain*: are the small-scale examples indicative of something bigger? The importance is not the size of a measurable effect, but what the data might indicate.

## Notes

1. Walter J. Rogan *et al.* 'Congenital poisoning by polychlorinated biphenyls and their contaminants in Taiwan', *Science* (1988), **241**, 334–6.

2. Theo Colborn *et al.*, *Our Stolen Future* (Little, Brown & Co.: London, 1996), p. 190.

3. Barbara Clayton, *Water Pollution at Lowermoor, North Cornwall* (HMSO: London, 1991), pp. 24–5.

4. Keith Schneider, 'Birth defects and pollution: issue raised in Texas town', *New York Times*, 15 April 1990, p. 14.

5. Guru Nandan, 'Brain damage found in victims of Bhopal disaster', *British Medical Journal* (1994), **308**, 359; Ingrid Eckerman, 'The health situation of women and children in Bhopal: final report of the Independent Medical Commission on Bhopal 1994', *International Perspectives on Public Health* (1996), **11** & **12**, 31.

6. Unpublished report of the '2nd Citizens Conference on Dioxins', at St Louis University, Tegler Hall, Missouri, 29–31 July 1994.

7. Colborn *et al.*, *op. cit.* (n. 2), p. 116.

8. Green Network. 'Baby food toxins', *Network News* (Green Network, Colchester, UK) (1995), Winter, 23.

9. John Elkington, *The Poisoned Womb* (Penguin: Harmondsworth, 1985), p. 21.

10. Lilo Altmann *et al.* 'Neurobehavioral and neurophysiological outcome of chronic low-level tetrachloroethene exposure measured in neighborhoods of dry cleaning shops', *Environmental Research* (1995), **69**, 83–9.

11. Nick Thorpe, 'A dirty story', *Observer*, 7 June 1992, pp. 40–6.

12. Mike Edwards, 'Lethal legacy', *National Geographic* (1994), **186**(2), 89.

13. Tara Patel, 'Rampant urban pollution blights Asia's crops', *New Scientist*, 14 June 1997, p 11.

14. L. Amin-Zaki *et al.*, 'Methylmercury poisoning in Iraqi children: clinical observations over two years', *British Medical Journal*, 11 March 1978, pp. 613–16.

15. A.E. Czeizel *et al.*, 'Environmental trichlorfon and cluster of congenital abnormalities', *The Lancet* (1993), **341**, 539–42.

16. Jane Seymour, 'Hungry for a new revolution', *New Scientist* (1996), **2023**, 32–7.

17. *Ibid.*, p. 34.

18. Patricia Sheenan and Irene B. Hillary, 'An unusual cluster of babies with Down's syndrome born to former pupils of an Irish boarding school', *British Medical Journal* (1983), **287**, 1428.

19. J.P. Bound, B.J. Francis and P.W. Harvey, 'Down's syndrome: prevalence and ionising radiation in an area of north west England', *Journal of Epidemiology and Community Health* (1995), **49**, 164–70.

20. Karl Sperling *et al.*, 'Significant increase in trisomy 21 in Berlin nine months after the Chernobyl reactor accident: temporal correlation or causal relation?', *British Medical Journal* (1994), **309**, 158–62; and letters, **309**, 1298–301.

21. Peter Bunyard, *Health Guide for the Nuclear Age* (Macmillan: London, 1988), p. 29.

22. Karl Sperling and Jorg Pelz, 'Authors stand by study that Chernobyl increased trisomy 21 in Berlin', *British Medical Journal* (1994), **309**, 1299.

23. David Marples, *The Social Impact of the Chernobyl Disaster* (St Martin's Press: New York, 1988), p. 44.

24. K.C. Johnson and J. Rouleau, *Tritium Releases from the Pickering Nuclear Generating Station and Birth Defects and Infant Mortality in Nearby Communities 1971-1988* (AECB project no. 7.156.1), and *Information Bulletin 91-3* (Atomic Energy Control Board: Ottawa, 1991), p. 4.

25. Tao Zufan and Wei Luxin, 'An epidemiological investigation of mutational diseases in the high background radiation area of Yangjiang, China', *Journal of Radiation Research* (1986), **27**, 151–62.

26. N. Kochupillai *et al.*, 'Down's syndrome and related abnormalities in an area of high background radiation in coastal Kerala', *Nature* (1976), **262**, 60–1.

27. *Sing Tao Daily*, May 1993, p. 15.

28. P.V. Unnikrishnan, 'Radiation – a ticking bomb', *Samadhan News* (Delhi) (1991), 5.

29. Madeleine Cobbing *et al.*, *Lead Astray: The Poisonous Lead Battery Trade* (Greenpeace: London, 1994).

30. Peter Lennon, 'Profits of doom on the border of blight', *Guardian*, 21 August 1992, p. 23.

31. UNICEF, *Global Child Health* (1993), **1**(2), 1. W.J. Rogan and B.C. Gladen, 'Breast feeding and cognitive development' *Early Human Development* (1993), **31**, 181–93.

32. K. Ghebremeskel *et al.*, 'Fatty acid composition of plasma and red cell phospholipids of preterm babies fed on breast milk and formulae', *European Journal of Pediatrics* (1995), **154**, 46–52.

33. C.R. Gale and C.N. Martyn, 'Breastfeeding, dummy use, and adult intelligence', *The Lancet* (1996), **347**, 1072–5.

34. *Ibid.*, p. 1027.

35. Des Wilson, *The Lead Scandal: The Fight to Save Children from Damage by Lead in Petrol* (Heinemann: London, 1983).

36. *Ibid.*, p. viii.

37. Peter H. Evans, 'The conioses: organic inflammatory oxidative responses to environmental particulate pollutants', in *Immunopharmacology of Free Radical Species* (Academic Press: London, 1995), p. 252.

38. Ministry of Public Health, Kuwait, *The Causes of Childhood Injury* (Ministry of Public Health; Al Jarah, 1985).

39. Rob Edwards, 'Smog blights babies in the womb', *New Scientist*, 19 October, 1996, p 4.

40. *Öko-bilanz eines Autolebens* (Umwelt- und Prognose-Institut Heidelberg: Landstrasse 118a, D-69121 Heidelberg, Germany, 1993).

41. Barry Hugill, 'Battery-hen children put on the fast lane to trouble', *Observer*, 25 July 1993, p. 57.

42. Robert Benson, 'Lead pollution from electric cars? Look a little closer at the facts', *Christian Science Monitor* (1995), **87**, 136.

43. Caroline Scott, 'A day in the life of Christina Noble', *Sunday Times Magazine*, 3 May 1994, p. 78.

44. Françoise Barten, *Environmental Lead Exposure of Children in Managua, Nicaragua* (CIP-Gegevens Koninklijke Bibliotheek: The Hague, 1992), p. viii.

45. A. Rimmer, 'Secret horror of a city called 19', *Sunday Mirror* (UK), 20 February 1994, pp. 12–13.

46. NRC, *Health Effects of Exposure to Low Levels of Ionizing Radiation* (BEIR V) (National Academy Press: Washington, DC, 1990).

47. E.R. Sternglass, 'The death of all children', *Esquire Magazine*, 1969, quoted in Rosalie Bertelle, *No Immediate Danger* (Women's Press: London, 1985), p. 231.

48. Carole Gallagher, *American Ground Zero: The Secret Nuclear War* (MIT Press: Cambridge, MA, 1993), p. 162.

49. Owen Dyer, 'Study links low dose radiation and Down's syndrome', *British Medical Journal* (1995), **310**, 1088–9. Full report in *Journal of Epidemiology and Community Health* (1995), **49**, 164–70.

50. M. De Andreis and F. Calogero, *The Soviet Nuclear Weapon Legacy* (Oxford University Press: Oxford, 1995).

51. C. Field, 'Child martyrs of Germany's own Chernobyl', *Observer*, 16 May 1993, p. 20.

52. D. Dembo, W. Morehouse and L. Wykle, *Abuse of Power* (New Horizons Press: New York, 1990), p. 40.

53. Elkington, *op. cit.* (n. 9), p. 215.

54. Joanna Ryan with Frank Thomas, *The Politics of Mental Handicap* (Churchill Livingstone: London, 1987).

# CHAPTER 7

# Pervasive Threats: Poverty, Nutrition and Health

If you are in Japan with $5 to spare, you can treat yourself to a three-pack of tuna eyeballs. Why tuna eyes come in threes is a mystery, but the reason that Japanese people eat something that tastes and looks so utterly revolting is not. The craze arose because of research suggesting that docosahexaenoic acid found in the eyeballs may help to improve brain performance. The acid is also added to other foodstuffs – including dog food. In 1992 a UK company was fined for marketing an 'IQ drug', which gave the false impression that it improved children's intelligence. On a grander scale in California, it was claimed in 1991 that a dietary supplement of vitamins and minerals had improved the achievement of over a million school children – children whose existing nutritional status was not clinically deficient.

> Move over Thomas Edison: make room for Yoshiro Nakamatsu, or Dr NakaMats as he is more pithily known. The good doctor is holder of more patents than anyone else, alive or dead . . . He presents a mug of Dr NakaMats 'brain tea' and proffers intelligence-enhancing Dr NakaMats Yummi Nutri Brain Cookies. From the pleat of his trousers he produces a small camera with which he photographs every meal he eats so that he can check which food stimulates the best inventions. Among the inventions are . . . compact discs playing classical music and subliminal messages to make the listener more intelligent . . . many of his best ideas come on long under-water swims starving the brain of oxygen . . . Nakamatsu needs just four hours' sleep . . . just three hours in his bed and one in his patented Cerebrex chair.[1]

Brain enhancement is also a growth area in the publishing world. There are now numerous books claiming to show how intelligence can be improved through diet. The books are based on reasonable science, but what they generally explain is how to avoid micro-nutrient deficiencies that are unlikely to be suffered by anyone who can afford the books. In 1995, those reading *New Scientist* learned that people who diet display a decrease in mental performance, but the reason was not biological. Mike Green of the UK Institute of Food Research explained, 'Constant thinking about food means that dieters don't have enough mental processing capacity to deal with [other] tasks properly.'[2] If worrying about food impairs the intellect, what is happening among the world's poor? The question follows logically, the implications would be massive, but it seems unlikely that *New Scientist* will ever provide the answer because the poor are not high on scientific research agendas – nor are they customers for *New Scientist*.

Throughout the rich nations, brain foods, brain tonics and brain books are now readily available to people with forms of intelligence indicating that such aids may indeed be necessary. Yet in the poor nations, poverty prevents the purchase of basic foodstuffs and medicines needed to mitigate even the simplest causes of intellectual decline.

## Degenerative spirals

Health, poverty and nutrition are inextricably intertwined. Recent work from the Center on Hunger, Poverty and Nutrition at Tufts University, Massachusetts, now challenges the simple theories of a linear causal connection between malnutrition, brain damage and delayed intellectual development. The old model is replaced by one that recognizes the complex interplay between other factors, such as poverty, lethargy and withdrawal, minimal exploration of the environment, delayed physical growth and lowered expectations from adults because the child appears young. The conclusion is that appropriate intervention can have a significant effect.[3] It is not just that millions of people do not now get the basic nutrients necessary for proper brain development. They are also unknowingly exposed to the possible threats from a large and increasing range of artificial additives in junk foods, which are linked to an array of sub-clinical intellectual and behavioural problems.[4]

Cerebral malaria can cause intellectual disability, and is widespread in poorer countries. There is concern in India that this disease, which was previously limited to a few tribal and north-east areas, has now spread to metropolitan centres. The cerebral form has increased from 25 to 40 per cent of total malaria cases in a decade. The over-use of pesticides and medical drugs is leading to new strains of the disease which resist conventional treatment. Japanese B encephalitis, which causes mental retardation and behaviour disorders, is spread by a mosquito from pigs to children and is endemic in South-east Asia. Both exposure and availability of treatment relate to socio-economic status.

Another significant health aspect stems from HIV/AIDS. About one-third of adults and a half of children with AIDS will develop neurological impairments because of HIV-1 infection of the central nervous system. The outcome is a mental slowing, diminished cognition, perhaps reading problems and a diminished ability to do simple daily tasks.[5] The high profile of the AIDS label masks a form of intellectual decline which, in another guise, might be termed mental handicap. Strictly speaking, AIDS itself is not an environmental health problem. But when we look at where the infection is endemic, it is all too obvious that many of those suffering will also be within the poverty–malnutrition–health spiral. The cause of infection may be something as simple as a hospital re-using a syringe because there is no money for disposables.

Anaemia is estimated to affect between one-third of men and two-thirds of women in poorer countries, leading to iron deficiency causing poor concentration and diminished mental abilities. A stomach parasite affecting a fifth of the world's population, hookworm, contributes not only to iron deficiency but also to protein malnutrition, culminating in impaired cognitive and motor development. Hookworm brings up the broader question. The condition is widespread and potentially easy to combat, yet research to find an effective cure has been minimal. Hookworm is a problem of the poor nations, and research agendas are largely dictated by the rich nations. In 1995, the US government gave geneticist Robert Plomin $600,000 to search for genes related to high intelligence, which is almost certainly a futile quest.

One of the few studies of prevalence of intellectual disability from a poor-nation perspective is from Bangladesh. The results concerning mild retardation are most significant: prevalence in the lower socio-economic group is nearly three times that in the middle and upper groups.[6] But this pattern is not contrary to that in the rich nations. The message is that poverty is a major threat to the brain, whether you are poor in a rich nation or poor in a poor one.

Science alone does not reveal the degenerative spirals of life within poorer communities. In the 1960s, a widely cited piece of opportunistic research examined the brains of 19 Chilean children who had died accidentally. It found that, while the brains of well-nourished children were not different from those of children in rich nations, those of severely malnourished children had a reduction in brain cells of up to 60 per cent.[7] This was, of course, reported principally as an important clinical finding. But the significance is less in the scientific discovery, and more that the findings describe the difference in children living within one country. The cause is internal inequity, not just the rich nation/poor nation divide.

Another graphic example comes from Brazil. Here 44 million people, a third of the population, suffer from stunted growth, and reduced brain size is noted in some regions. In the words of one observer, 'Dwarfism diminishes the capacity to work, rationalize and intellectualize, which means that the person grows less, learns less and has less capacity for work.' This is not an impoverished nation – Brazil boasts that its economy is among the world's top ten.[8]

Even within countries like the UK, inequity can stem from an environmental cause. The increase in out-of-town superstores has caused the closure of many small local shops – a car is necessary to purchase even the most basic foods at a reasonable cost. The result is a significant level of nutrition-related developmental problems in children in inner-city areas such as Hackney, London. Urban environmental change can be as relevant as land degradation in relation to the availability of necessary foods to poor populations.

> Undernourishment and malnutrition account for a higher percentage of cases of intellectual retardation in children and suboptimal function in adults than all other causes put together.[9]

The link between poor nutrition and intellectual decline was established and acknowledged throughout the world by the start of the 1970s, yet the value of simple intervention is still being questioned. In a well-known study of remediation, children who suffered malnutrition in early life and were not helped ended up with IQs of 70, as compared to children with a similar condition who did receive help, who ended up with a near-normal average IQ of 99.[10] The realization is not just that poverty-related malnutrition causes the initial problem, but that a poverty-related absence of remediation can make it permanent.

One piece of research made the rich nation/poor nation contrast crystal-clear. This found that malnourished Korean orphans adopted by US families by the age of three had normal IQ scores by the age of 12; those not adopted did not. The cure was therefore not one of medical science – to live in an American household was sufficient. There is a further irony. In the rich nations, obese women are twice as likely to have babies with birth impairments, including anencephaly (absence of a brain).[11] Wealth-related over-consumption strikes at intellectual resources through many routes.

Like our knowledge of lead, our knowledge of the relationship between poor nutrition and intellectual development is well established. Despite this, it is easier to persuade an education ministry to fund a new curriculum change than to provide a school meals service, or vitamin and mineral pills that would cost no more than the equivalent of a few hours' tuition a year. Addressing the problems of children who for pedagogical reasons *do not* learn is much more attractive than addressing the problems of those who, for the sake of a daily bowl of soup, eventually *cannot* learn.

## Iatrogenicity

One of the most problematic and unrecognized synergisms in the poverty–health–nutrition spiral is iatrogenic effects – the cures that cause ills.

Many common clinical drugs are potentially neurotoxic,[12] so any general increase in environmental health problems, even if not directly affecting the brain, might increase the risk of iatrogenic brain damage. In the UK, among miners who were treated with aluminium powder to prevent silicotic lung disease, the outcome was a clear and dose-related decline in cognitive function.[13] There are less obvious synergisms. The over-use of antibiotics leads to vitamin deficiencies, which can cause *absence*-EMID. Add to this the problem of over-prescribing in some poorer countries, which can amount to 40 per cent, and modern clinical medicine can pose a significant threat to intellectual resources in some circumstances.

There is a well-established link between adverse environments and stress.[14] Drugs used to treat stress function by targeting, and often then by reducing, overall brain functioning. The tranquillizer Valium is known to have reduced the mental age of a British atomic scientist, Reg Peart, to 10. Even seven years after he stopped taking the drug, tests showed that he was still suffering a 20 per cent intellectual impairment.[15]

Hospital treatments are also problematic. Even simple operations have a small risk of brain damage from oxygen starvation while under a general anaesthetic. There is a fourfold increase in children born with Down's syndrome to mothers who have more than four X-rays prior to conception.[16] Ultrasound scans, especially new, more powerful forms such as Doppler scanning, are suspected of disrupting language development. Dentistry is thought to pose a hazard because of mercury from amalgam fillings entering the blood. Children from poorer families inevitably have many more fillings (if dental treatment is available). Studies in the USA and Germany have linked Alzheimer's disease with mercury fillings, and the levels of mercury in babies correlate with the number of amalgam fillings their mothers have. The Swedish government has prohibited the use of mercury fillings in children under 12 and is considering a complete ban from 1997. Because mercury crosses the placenta, their use for women between 15 and 50 is likely to be prohibited in Germany. But the governments of less wealthy nations (which include Britain) maintain that there is no risk. Mercury may also constitute a potential occupational health hazard to dentists and technicians. Amalgam fillings may well eventually be banned through occupational health legislation, not because of the risk to patients. Fluoridation of water, intended to improve dental health, is linked to Down's syndrome. Russian studies in the 1970s found that fluoride impaired mental functioning, but these findings were ignored by Western policy-makers.[17]

Perhaps most significant are the iatrogenic effects on the unborn child. The consequences of the drug thalidomide finally persuaded the medical world that the human placenta does not protect from all chemical insults – a possibility that had been indicated by animal experiments for many years. The image associated with thalidomide is of physical impairments, but the drug also caused brain impairment, including autism, if it was used at a particular point in foetal development. One of the most important lessons from thalidomide is that the US Food and Drugs Agency operated the 'precautionary principle' and the drug was never licensed for use in the USA, sparing millions its impact.

Intellectual disability caused by childhood vaccination became such a contentious issue in the UK that special legislation was introduced to deal with compensation claims.[18] Despite the hurdles put up to deter compensation (see Chapter 11), over 800 UK children are formally recognized as victims of whooping cough vaccine.

Little has changed over time. Vaccination for measles, mumps and rubella introduced in 1988 was withdrawn in 1992 because of a risk of meningitis. A Department of Health leaflet promoted the vaccine as preventing brain damage through disease, but did not mention that brain damage could be a side-effect. Why were vaccines used in the UK that had been banned in Japan, never used in the USA and withdrawn two years earlier in Canada?

All vaccinations contain formaldehyde, aluminium phosphate and a mercury compound, thiomersal, which are potentially hazardous to the brain. The dynamics of globalization and the probable increase in communicable disease, particularly if fuelled further by global warming and other environmental change, will precipitate a greater use of vaccines. Inevitably the poorer countries will use the cheaper but more dangerous types (no doubt enthusiastically promoted and supplied by rich-nation pharmaceutical companies); the iatrogenic threat to the human brain will inevitably increase.

Iatrogenic hazards are not all of Western origin. Some traditional Indian cures dispensed by ethnic practitioners or *hakim*, such as those used to treat eczema, contain mercury levels that are highly neurotoxic.[19] Occasionally, traditional Chinese medicine practised in the UK has caused damage to the central nervous system, and raw herbs used to make the remedies are sometimes contaminated with heavy metals and pesticides. Other traditional treatments embody a more obvious environmental cause; for example, cod-liver oil, often used in the care of pregnant women, sometimes now contains hazardous levels of PCBs or mercury. In India the use of treatments banned in the West – oestrogen and progesterone drugs, for example – is clearly linked to brain impairment and other birth disabilities. It is well within the power of the Indian government to ban their use.

The cures that cause ills are not always directly medical. The US Environmental Protection Agency is concerned about the use of insect repellants containing diethyltoluamide, to protect from tick-borne bacteria which cause Lyme disease. Excessive application has caused intellectual impairment in children. On a larger scale, the over-use of insecticides has led to insects becoming immune to these chemicals. Mosquitoes are a particular concern because their modified metabolism creates drug-resistant forms of cerebral malaria and resultant brain damage.

The case of tuberculosis (TB) perhaps best exemplifies the iatrogenic spirals surrounding EMID. TB in children, a disease related to a poor environment, can itself cause intellectual disability. But intellectual disability can also be one of the side-effects of drug treatment – particularly the cheaper drugs that are used within poorer communities. In India it is not unusual to be told of 'whole villages with TB'. But more experienced doctors will often correct this to 'whole villages *are being treated for* TB'. Why? Because in its early stages TB has similar symptoms to numerous other poverty-related diseases. Inexperienced doctors often prefer to take no chances and treat any condition with TB-like symptoms as TB. Perhaps intent is benign, but some Indian doctors will mention the benefits to their colleagues. TB treatment takes many months and entails considerable expenditure on drugs. This creates a reliable source of fees, and possibly commissions for promoting drug use, for young, badly paid doctors. In communities with low intellectual resources, the knowledge and ability to challenge exploitation of this nature is increasingly limited, and the degenerative spiral is perpetuated.

As so often in relation to EMID, the most overlooked aspect of iatrogenicity is the perspective of those with an existing intellectual disability. Clinical drugs used in relation to intellectual disability sometimes increase the disability.[20] Epilepsy commonly accompanies other brain impairments, and this is often treated with phenobarbitone, which further depresses intellectual functioning. Some of the drugs used to control aggressive behaviour do this by reducing overall brain functioning. The temptation to use these drugs, as opposed to other forms of highly skilled labour-intensive intervention, is great because of the cost saving. The use of Ritalin to make children who suffer from attention deficit hyperactivity disorder more obedient and attentive at school was eventually questioned by parents, because the side-effects include a loss of zest and personality, creating 'zombie-like' children. The combination of modern medical zeal and social pressures makes it so very easy to indulge in cures that do little more than impose an intellectual disability on a behavioural disability.

It is easy to lose the thread that connects health, iatrogenicity, EMID and environmental change. Leukaemia caused by radiation exemplifies the links. The cause can be environmental – nuclear waste, for instance. Leukaemia does not directly threaten the brain, but the cures do. Not only is chemotherapy treatment for leukaemia potentially neurotoxic, but some forms of radiation treatment used to cure cancers can also lead to brain impairment. What was the root cause of the brain impairment – the treatment or the pollution?

The risk of iatrogenic effects must, of course, be balanced by the potential of medicine to mitigate the threats to the brain and to health generally. But the point is not that we need yet more research to see if the benefits of medicine outweigh the risks of treatment, but that without the environmental hazards we would not need to do this research. The iatrogenic threat results fundamentally from environmental, not medical, ills. In some settings *most* disease now stems from an environmental cause – 80 per cent if you live in the former USSR.

## Alcohol and drugs misuse

The misuse of alcohol and drugs is not often perceived as an environmental problem. But it is technological change that has made potentially harmful substances so widely available in recent years. In the case of alcohol and tobacco, this is compounded by pervasive forms of advertising that are now part of our everyday environment. The environmental conceptualization is most persuasive from the perspective of the unborn child. Increasingly the mobile environment of the baby – its mother – is as polluted as any city.

It is not disputed that recreational drugs and other substance abuse directly affect the brain – that is precisely what these chemicals are designed to do. The question is whether or not brain impairment becomes permanent, and the real hazard is that no one knows. The drug ecstasy (MDMA) has attracted recent interest, and it is now known to cause permanent brain impairment in rodents and monkeys at dose levels comparable with human use. Accidental human ingestion of a related substance (MPTP) caused severe and irreversible effects.[21] Another study suggests that ecstasy users may eventually lose serotonin function and become more susceptible to memory loss and dementia.[22] The scale of the potential threat seems unlikely to diminish. Ten per cent of 14- to 19-year-olds in the UK use ecstasy. Even conservative predictions from the British police conclude that 70 to

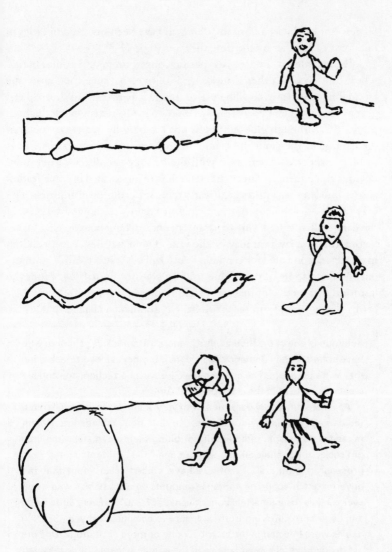

'When I'm smoking the glue I get very scared. Many things are coming to get me; the cars and the big snake. It wants to eat me. There is also the BIG hole. It wants to swallow me. I run, but it is difficult to get away.'

(Saul, aged 12)

**Figure 7.1** 'What I see in my head when I sniff glue'.
*Source:* Christopher Williams, 'Street children and education', PhD thesis, University of Birmingham (1990).

80 per cent of children born in 1996 'will have been involved in drugs in one form or another by the time they are 10 or 11'.[23]

Solvent abuse by children is a specific concern in poorer communities, where the cost of other drugs is prohibitive, because they cross the blood–brain barrier easily. The use of thinners, benzene and shoemakers' glue by street children has become a common media stereotype throughout the world. Although glue sniffing is not biologically addictive, much of the damage to the brain and central nervous system is irreversible. But as so often happens, a fascination with the biology can distract from more obvious consequences. Street children who are intoxicated become fearless and commonly run in front of cars, then suffering head injuries. The drawing by a Johannesburg street child in Figure 7.1 shows awareness of the danger. If you are trying to escape an encroaching hole or a big snake, getting run over by a car may be the least of your worries. Street children have been documented for centuries – 'blackguards', 'street arabs', 'gamin' – but the first report of them glue sniffing was not until 1964. From the historical perspective of the street child tradition, this new threat to their brains clearly stems from recent global environmental change.[24]

> Solomon is one of the thousands of American 'crack kids', children who have suffered brain damage because their mothers smoked crack when they were pregnant. The children have just reached school age and are creating mayhem in the classrooms of America.
>
> A few are physically deformed, with very small heads, but more often the damage is less obvious. Some, like Solomon, explode into violent rages for no reason, often kicking or biting their playmates. One little girl rocks in her chair all day without speaking . . . Some states have prosecuted mothers . . . others have voiced resentment that the government is 'spending immense amounts on crack babies who won't ever achieve the intellectual consciousness of God' . . . Every 90 seconds a baby is born suffering from exposure to cocaine. Last year, 375,000 babies were infected in the womb by one or more illicit drugs. Doctors are divided over the permanence of the damage; there is little research on the problem because it is so new.[25]

Because widespread drugs use is relatively new, the nature of the threat to the brain of the unborn child is less well established than in relation to smoking. It is known that solvents cross the placenta and a syndrome nearly identical to that caused by alcohol has been identified in children of mothers who sniffed toluene during pregnancy. Sub-clinical outcomes include attention deficit and developmental delays. Gasoline inhalation by the mother is linked to mental retardation in the child, but this might be due to its lead content. Without question, hard drugs pose a problem.

Unfortunately the response has been to punish mothers rather than to prevent and mitigate the fundamental problems through appropriate social support.[26] This culminates in mothers at risk not seeking medical help, which furthers the risk to their unborn children. Merrill Berger of the Children's Hospital in Boston tells how, 'the day after a mother was charged with "distributing" cocaine to her foetus (the infant had tested positive for cocaine), the clinic, usually fully booked, was nearly empty'.[27]

Not only is the punitive response counterproductive, it is also unjust if women are perceived as the only concern. Male-mediated effects are also possible. Dr Wylie Hembry of Columbia University has found that heavy marijuana smoking can reduce sperm count and increase the numbers of abnormally shaped sperm. He elaborates:

> Marijuana may be one of many environmental agents that affect sperm development, not enough to make you sterile but enough to have subtle harmful effects on subsequent generations, so subtle that we don't yet know how to monitor them. This is more worrisome than if marijuana made men sterile.[28]

It is probably scientific inadequacy, not biological fact, that currently presents women as the main culprits concerning drug-related reproductive threats to the brains of unborn children.

The link between women smoking and developmental deficits in their babies, principally because of low birth weight, is well established. In many countries cigarette advertising now carries a warning (Figure 7.2). Consequences for infants include smaller head size, and neurobehavioural deficits such as impaired psychomotor development, decreased auditory responsiveness and poorer orientation and attention spans.[29] Smoking also seems to precipitate EMID in unborn children through causing nutritional deficits and increasing the uptake of heavy metals. Put more simply, if you pollute the mobile environment of the baby and its brain through smoking, it seems that it is then less able to cope with the threats posed by the external environment.

But again the preoccupation with pregnant women can be misleading. An increase in mental retardation among children whose fathers smoked cigars or pipes at the time of birth was found by a Dutch study, perhaps caused by sperm damage or the passive smoking by mothers.[30]

There is considerable evidence that smoking is a cause of diseases that can contribute directly to brain damage. Nicotine is a natural pesticide, used by the tobacco plant to deter predators by injuring their nervous

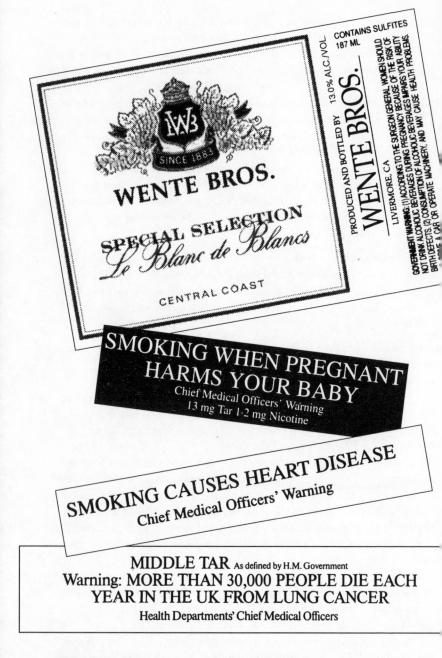

**Figure 7.2**  Statutory warnings on alcohol and cigarettes.

system. It is not therefore surprising that there is an adverse impact on the human brain.

Direct brain damage to adults from alcohol is also well established. High alcohol intake shrinks the substance of the brain. At the severe end of the scale the effect appears largely irreversible. Although not killing brain cells, as was originally thought, excess alcohol damages nerve pathways. Sub-clinical effects include a decline in memory and non-verbal cognitive skills.[31] Alcohol abuse causes vitamin deficiencies, especially of thiamine, and the effects on the brain have been known for a century. Chronic alcoholism is the commonest cause of malnutrition in the developed world because alcohol mimics nutrients and the body then rejects the real thing.[32] Little thought has been given to cumulative decline caused by alcohol, which may become significant in old age.

As with drugs misuse, the threat to the unborn child is significant. And in some countries there are now statutory warnings to this effect (Figure 7.2). Foetal alcohol syndrome (FAS) is now stated to be the 'leading known cause of mental retardation' in the USA.[33] Between 2 and 8 per cent of children born to alcoholic women will suffer intellectual disability. Women who consume a typical seven drinks a week tend to concentrate consumption over two or three days, which can impair brain function in their babies if it happens at a particular time in gestation.[34] Less acute foetal alcohol effects (FAE) include reduced habituation and delayed language development, and impacts may be compounded by poverty and malnutrition.

Alcohol problems among indigenous peoples who have suffered because of colonial and neo-colonial exploitation provide a media stereotype, which is rarely adequately explained. The blame-the-victim spiral set up by images of 'drunken aboriginals' sometimes masks a greater problem – high levels of FAS. The rate among American Indian children is 33 times higher than among non-Indians. The degenerative spiral might, in the case of North American fishing communities, such as the Cree, be furthered by the ingestion of mercury from contaminated fish. Both problems, from the perspective of those affected, are, of course, a product of colonial intrusion.

In microcosm, substance abuse epitomizes the social dynamics of EMID. Human behaviour and cultural forces are the key, not the nature of chemicals. Poverty plays its part. There is apparent choice, but not for the unborn child. Research and remedy are dictated by politics (in this case the politics of morality), and broader political forces dictate the overall circumstance. Cumulative and synergistic effects are very probable, but unresearched.

The exponential increase and unpredictable nature of substance dependency and alcohol abuse are one of the biggest experiments with its intellectual resources that humankind has ever conducted. And in the context of millions of years of human brain evolution, it is a very recent experiment.

## Notes

1. Kevin Rafferty, 'Patents are a virtue but not in Japan', *Observer*, 25 February 1996, p. 7.

2. 'Memory loss by inches', *Down to Earth* (India) (1995), **4**(15), 46.

3. J. Larry Brown and Ernesto Pollitt, 'Malnutrition, poverty and intellectual development', *Scientific American* (1996), **274**(2), 26–31.

4. C.B. Travis *et al.*, *Environmental Toxins: Psychological, Behavioral, and Sociocultural Aspects, 1973–1989* (American Psychological Association: Washington, DC, 1989), pp. 85–92.

5. Hans S.L.M. Nottet, 'Unravelling the neuroimmune mechanisms for the HIV-1-associated cognitive/motor complex', *Immunology Today* (1995), **16**(9), 441–8.

6. S. Islam, M. Durkin and S.S. Zaman, 'Socioeconomic status and the prevalence of mental retardation in Bangladesh', *Mental Retardation* (1993), **31**(6), 412–17.

7. M. Winick and P. Rosso, 'Head circumference and cellular growth of the brain in normal and marasmic children', *Journal of Pediatrics* (1969), **74**, 774.

8. Louis Byrne, 'Crippling poverty stunts Brazilian growth', *Observer*, 26 January 1992, p. 12.

9. R. Sterner, *Social and Economic Conditions of the Mentally Retarded in Selected Countries* (UN/ILSMH: Brussels, 1976).

10. H.P. Chase and N.P. Martin, 'Undernutrition and child development', *New England Journal of Medicine* (1975), **282**, 933–9.

11. P. Cohen, 'Overweight mums put babies at risk', *New Scientist* (1996), **2026**, 8.

12. P. Jenner and C.D. Marsden, 'Neurological toxicity of drugs', in J.W. Gorrod (ed.), *Drug Toxicity* (Taylor & Francis: London, 1979), pp. 151–8.

13. S.L. Rifat *et al.* 'Effect of exposure of miners to aluminium powder', *The Lancet* (1990), **336**, 1162–5.

14. Gary W. Evans, *Environmental Stress* (Cambridge University Press: Cambridge, 1982).

15. Patricia Davies, 'Doctors dished them out like sweets until, like opium, they got the masses hooked', *Independent*, 19 August 1996, p. 6.

16. B.B. Oppenhelm *et al.*, 'The effects of diagnostic x-ray on the human foetus: an examination of the evidence', *Radiology* (1975), **114**, 529–34.

17. Bob Woffinden, 'Clear and present danger', *Guardian Weekend*, 7 June 1997, pp. 27–30.

18. Vaccine Damage Payments Act 1979 (UK).

19. John Kew *et al.*, 'Arsenic and mercury intoxication due to Indian ethnic remedies', *British Medical Journal* (1993), **306**, 506–7.

20. Solomon H. Snyder, *Drugs and the Brain* (Macmillan Press: Basingstoke, 1996).

21. A.R. Green and G.M. Goodwin, 'Ecstasy and neurodegeneration', *British Medical Journal* (1996), **312**, 1493.

22. Oliver James, 'Ecstasy has sown mental illness seed,' *Observer*, 15 December 1996, p. 3.

23. David Brindle, 'Drugs fear for under-11s', *Guardian*, 31 January 1996, p. 2.

24. Uwe von Dücker, 'Drogen-, Alkohol- und Lösungsmittelmißbrauch bei lateinamerikanischen Straßenkindern', *Rundbrief* (1964), **2**, 28–35.

25. G. Greig, 'Crack kids give America a new lesson in suffering', *Sunday Times*, 8 March 1992, p. 21.

26. L.S. Welch, 'Organic solvents' (Chapter 19) and H.W. Clarke and M. Weinstein, 'Chemical dependency' (Chapter 25), in M. Paul (ed.), *Occupational and Environmental Reproductive Hazards: A Guide for Clinicians* (Williams & Wilkins: Baltimore, 1993)

27. Merrill Berger, 'Behind bars before birth', *Observer*, 18 August 1991, p. 44.

28. Jane Brody, 'Sperm found especially vulnerable to environment', *New York Times (Science Times)*, 10 March 1981, p. C1.

29. H.W. Clark and M. Weinstein, 'Chemical dependency', in M. Paul (ed.), *Occupational and Environmental Reproductive Hazards: A Guide for Clinicians* (Williams & Wilkins: Baltimore, 1993), pp. 347–8.

30. Nel Roeleveld *et al.*, 'Mental retardation associated with parental smoking and alcohol consumption before, during, and after pregnancy', *Preventive Medicine* (1992), **21**, 110–19.

31. A.D. Thomson *et al.*, 'Alcohol and brain damage', *Human Toxicology* (1988), **7**, 455–63.

32. G.K. Shaw, *The Last Ten Years of Research, Elmdene Alcohol Unit* (bibliography) (London: The Brain Damage Research Trust, 1990).

33. Berger, *op. cit.* (n. 27).

34. Abraham Rosenberg, 'Brain damage caused by prenatal alcohol exposure', *Science & Medicine* (1996), **3**(4), 42–51.

# CHAPTER 8

# The Cure?

Whether from research or common sense and observation, there is now a growing recognition of EMID in its many forms. What is the practical response? One aspect is curious. Although EMID is relevant to both health and education policy, it is only within health that a clear strategy can be identified. There is conclusive evidence demonstrating that EMID can have a general effect on the behaviour and learning ability of schoolchildren, and in specific cases it is known to have significant effects. But there is almost no recognition of this through the adaptation of teaching approaches or development of teacher attitudes.

## Health

The glossy brochure from the Foundation for Children of the Copper Basin in Legnica in Poland might be taken for the type of publicity material used by thousands of education projects, schools and children's non-governmental organizations (NGOs) worldwide. The photos show smiling children engaged in rural pursuits and dedicated staff who set up the foundation in 1991. But the graphs inside do not depict exam success or attendance figures. They show the level of lead poisoning in children in relation to their proximity to copper smelters, and the results of detox treatment. Therapy includes a diet of mineral-rich water which 'competes' with the heavy metals, bee products and special exercise. But unfortunately, when treated, the children return to the polluted towns that caused their initial problems.

A similar strategy is employed to help the survivors of the nuclear power disaster at Chernobyl. Dr Zolovok of the Children's Hospital in Soligork claims that 'Just a month of fresh food, clean air, and vitamins, greatly boosts their immune systems.' Following the poisoning of nine million people by polybrominated biphenyls (PBBs) by the Michigan Chemical Corporation, the Foundation for Advancements in Science and Education in Los Angeles devised a remediation programme involving exercise, sauna and diet, and the use of niacin to detoxify the body. The reduction of body burdens of

PBBs by about 25 per cent resulted in an improvement in reaction times by 20 per cent and long-term memory by over 15 per cent.[1]

Non-Western approaches display a degree more sophistication. In 1995, it was reported that Indian scientists had found that traditional Ayurvedic cures are an effective treatment for heavy metal and other environmental poisoning.[2] Dr S. K. Dwivedi of the Indian Veterinary Research Institute in Izatnagar describes how pomegranate juice, a mixture of radish and soya seed, a drink of milk with sugar, or lemon juice with sugar can be used to treat lead poisoning. *Withania somnifera* (aswagandha) appears an effective treatment for poisoning by lead, mercury and iodine because its roots have a sedative effect. Black gram, grapes and carrots seem to counter the sub-clinical effects of continuous low-level exposure to heavy metals. Other herbal remedies contain vitamins and minerals that counter the take-up of heavy metals.

The Environmental Unit at Brookhaven Hospital, set up by Dr William Rea, is the high-tech version of clinical ecology. It is completely sealed, and constructed only of inert materials such as tiles, metals and stone. The air is circulated over charcoal filters to remove stray chemicals. For those especially allergic to modern environmental chemicals, the unit provides the only means to a reasonable life.

In Worcester, Massachusetts, the Occupational and Reproductive Hazards Center goes a stage further than basic health remediation, recognizing the social justice perspective. Through outreach programmes operating in English and Spanish, some specifically targeted at immigrant workers, the centre not only assesses occupational hazards and medical care, but can also address legal issues. It contributes to state policy decisions on environmental pollution and occupational hazards. The strength of this approach is that it is not just a cure for an immediate problem, but a route to improved prevention which is better informed because of grass-roots involvement. This is important because otherwise remediation simply becomes a palliative minimizing problems that should not be permitted to arise in the first place.

On the preventive side, many US states now screen children routinely for lead and other heavy metals. Massachusetts tests around a half of those under 6. In the context of the long-standing knowledge about lead, it is remarkable to find a modern country such as France suddenly waking up to its lead problem, and finding that 10 per cent of a sample of Parisian children suffered poisoning. In 1994, a US$8 million budget was made available to deal with the problem.[3] The main cause was lead in house dust and old paintwork. Lead in paint was banned in 1948, since when it had been assumed that the problem had been solved. The involvement of Médecins sans Frontières, an organization usually associated with international disaster relief, to provide a solution suggests a degree of urgency.

A few decades ago these reports would have seemed like science fiction; in a few decades' time they may represent a norm in polluted regions. The interest is the similarity of approach, which is not highly sophisticated, but usually relies on removing those affected from the toxic threat, providing a diet of basic natural foods that address the bodily synergisms that can worsen or precipitate the effects of environmental toxins, and simple detox techniques. The cure, like the cause, is mainly environmental. Will this approach become more central to medicine? With a sixth of American children as the potential market, how long before the carrot is patented as a cure for low-level lead poisoning?

## Education

Anywhere in the world there are two complaints within schools: unsatisfactory educational achievement and behaviour problems. And it is easy to see the link. Within schools in their current form, low-achieving pupils are less likely to behave appropriately; those who do not behave appropriately are less likely to achieve their educational potential. It is also easy to see the possible links between the known effects of environmental chemicals on the brain and these two school problems. But despite a wealth of evidence concerning effects on populations, definitive proof in relation to individuals seems elusive, so the possibility never becomes a probability in the minds of educationalists.

The American Psychological Association publishes a bibliography, *Environmental Toxins: Psychological, Behavioral, and Sociocultural Aspects*, which lists nearly one thousand papers.[4] Can they all be meaningless? Would scientists have spent so much time in this area if there were no credibility in the findings? In the light of this weight of evidence, how often does the schoolteacher look at a class whose behaviour is problematic and whose achievement is unsatisfactory, and even give a thought that the cause might, in some part, be our modern chemical environment? Perhaps in places such as Legnica teachers now do so.

Many chemicals known to affect individual behaviour seem not to have widespread effects across whole populations. But they do have significant effects on a small percentage within those populations. The link between particular food additives and the behaviour of particular children is one of the key examples. And, in the light of what we know of schools, it is interesting to note that boys seem to be more at risk from this particular impact than girls.

But this should not lead us to the conclusion that the total effect of environmental chemicals on school life is therefore marginal – we just do not know. We know that some substances such as lead and mercury *do* have a widespread effect on those exposed. And we know that populations are exposed to thousands of artificial substances, most untested for their impact on the brain. To this can be added the likelihood that mixtures of environmental chemicals may be producing other, completely unrecognized outcomes. What then of *absence*-EMID, which is largely but not exclusively a poor-nation problem? The cumulative outcome of EMID within schools could now be significant, but it will not be immediately apparent to teachers who just accept the behaviour and achievement levels they find as an undesirable norm.

Rarely does teacher education include *any* consideration of the standard scientific literature concerning the relationship between environmental chemicals, and behaviour and achievement. Is this because there is no value in doing so, because of tradition or because the political desire to deny EMID influences training institutions? Teacher education is, after all, always in the control of governments.

From a teacher's perspective, one of the most convincing pieces of research came from Herbert Needleman in the USA, in 1979.[5] This concerned over 3000 children. The results were then replicated in the UK by William Yule and Richard Lansdown,[6] and no serious fault has been found with these studies since. There are now numerous similar findings. Needleman simply asked teachers to rank pupils in relation to the following headings, and few teachers would disagree that this list reflects what is problematic about their daily work. Pupils are:

- distractible

- not persistent

- dependent

- not organized

- hyperactive

- impulsive

- frustrated

- day-dreamers

- unable to follow simple directions

- unable to follow sequences

- low functioning overall

The result of the two studies was that the teachers' perception of these problems related directly to the levels of lead in their pupils' teeth, and that IQ deficits in individual children also fitted the overall pattern. This is about as near as any piece of research could ever get to demonstrating beyond doubt that an environmental chemical causes some of the behaviour and achievement problems that so bedevil schools. And remember that in the USA, this might relate to a sixth of all children; in some African cities 90 per cent.

Needleman did not leave his findings at this point, and in 1988 he revisited work he had done between 1975 and 1978.[7] He discovered that children with high lead levels in their teeth when they were aged 6 and 7 displayed 'a markedly higher risk of dropping out of high school . . . lower class standing in high school, increased absenteeism, lower vocabulary and grammatical-reasoning scores'. 'For the small group of 10 subjects who were diagnosed earlier as having plumbism, the outcome was especially dire; half these people have reading disabilities, and almost half left school before graduation.' Needleman concluded with something of an under-statement: 'exposure to lead, even in children who remain asymptomatic, may have an enduring effect on the success of such children . . . the implications of these findings for attempts to prevent school failure are intriguing.' Put another way: new curricula, codes of discipline, textbooks and innovative teaching methods, while not unimportant, are of *secondary* importance when children have suffered even mild exposure to a neurotoxin.

In the area of *presence*-EMID, only lead has attracted sufficient attention to provide such conclusive results, but these findings are almost certainly applicable to many other neurotoxins. Remember that in the Czech Republic and Poland there is a belief that pollution is now responsible for doubling the need for special education places in schools. And this conclusion is only in relation to children clearly seen as having problems; it indicates a much larger level of sub-clinical intellectual decline throughout the school population generally. More recent concern about the effects of hormone-disrupting chemicals reflects the lead story. In time we could see similar conclusions which may be even more concerning because of the persistence in the body of the chemicals involved – the detox remedy is much more problematic (see Appendix).

The outcome of *absence*-EMID within schools in the poorer nations is even less well researched, perhaps because the children affected will drop out of school or never enrol, so to the teacher the circumstance is a self-solving problem. The reported efficacy of iodization programmes suggests the impact of iodine deficiency on schools. As a result of iodized oil injections in Ecuador,

Why did the Scholastic Aptitude Test scores of high school seniors seeking college admission begin to fall sharply from their high point in 1963 and continue downwards for almost two decades? . . . What about the problems in our schools? Why can't many children read? Is it because they watch too much TV or spend all their time playing video games, because of a lack of family support for schools, or because they were exposed to PCBs or other thyroid-disrupting chemicals before birth?

While any connection is still speculative, the human and animal studies reporting learning difficulties and hyperactivity in those exposed prenatally to PCBs suggest to us that synthetic chemicals may indeed be increasing the burden on our schools . . . save for lead and mercury, educators, physicians, and others have been slow to recognize that the chemical environment may undermine educational efforts as well as social environment.[8]

*Scholastic achievement was better in the children of treated mothers when measured in terms of school year reached for age, school drop-out rate, failure rate, years repeated, and school marks . . . Both groups were impaired in school performance, in reading, writing, and mathematics, but more notably the children of untreated mothers.*[9]

In most rich nations all newborn children are checked for the level of thyroid hormones, and thyroxine is given to correct any deficiency. IQ is severely affected if the treatment is not available within the first three months. In the poorer countries where the problem is greatest, universal screening does not happen.

If prevention is inadequate, mitigation should be a priority. Surely in a country such as Bhutan, where iodine deficiency is known to affect the intelligence of 22 per cent of the population, educational policy and teaching techniques should reflect this problem. The reason why education ministries do not respond is almost certainly that the relevant data are locked in the domain of health ministries, and those officials able to bring relevant ministries together will not put the problem on the agenda because of the possible economic and political ramifications.

Even the most basic facts are rarely imparted to teachers as part of their training. Experiments assessing the take-up of radioactive glucose by the brain have now demonstrated that the brains of people of low intelligence measurably consume more energy than those of greater intelligence when solving the same problems. Children who suffer intellectual decline because of protein–energy malnutrition will therefore need *more* energy than their more fortunate peers to achieve the same results. The degenerative spiral is not hard to envisage, yet awareness of simple biological problems of this nature is rare among teachers in poorer countries, who are supposed to have received a training appropriate to the circumstances of the communities in which they will work.

We know the fundamental solutions to nutritional deficiencies, but they are not applied effectively. India's midday meals scheme is well-intentioned, but corruption and mismanagement often lead to meals that are said to contain more neurotoxins than nutrients. Ingredients are stolen, meals are watered down and the aluminium from the cooking pots pollutes the food, as do toxins from chemical cleaning agents. This could be remedied, but in the meantime teachers could at least be a little more accommodating of the intellectual problems that political and social neglect causes children.

> Inadequate nutrition can disrupt cognition – although in different ways than were previously assumed. At one time, underfeeding in childhood was thought to hinder mental development solely by producing permanent, structural damage to the brain. More recent work, however, indicates that malnutrition can impair the intellect by other means as well . . . These new findings have important implications for policies aimed at bolstering achievement among underprivileged children.
>
> . . . although schools can provide much of the stimulation children need, early malnutrition can undermine the overall value of education . . . The US invests billions of dollars in education, yet much of this money goes to waste when children appear at the school door intellectually crippled from undernutrition.[10]

What changes in education policy and practice could reasonably be expected in response to EMID and related behaviour problems? Principally, the approach to education will need to embrace a broader 'special needs' approach across a whole school. It is now not adequate to assume that most children can learn through the standard class methods, be they labelled traditional or progressive. More attention will need to be paid to developmental skills – cognitive, spatial, perceptional. This must go beyond simply trying to redress an apparent intellectual deficit. A knowledge of the effects of specific forms of EMID will become necessary; for example, reflecting the fact that some chemical exposures have a particular effect on adaptive skills. The knowledge that extensive car use diminishes children's coping and social skills provides a clear deficit that schools in rich nations should now address.

Special schools will need to adapt to a new clientele. At the Teddy de Souza Learning Center in New York, which originally catered only for children with traditional forms of intellectual and physical disability, more than half the pupils are now the 'crack kids' who suffer intellectual and behavioural problems because their mothers abused drugs during pregnancy. Like much of what is now mainstream educational practice, general education innovation may well stem from these specialist institutions. At a centre for young offenders in Cumbria, UK, the director, Bernard Gesch, treats those in his charge with wholefood diets and vitamin supplements because, even without direct clinical proof, he believes that this has an impact on behaviour.

The current environmental impact on learning does not just involve direct effects on the brain, and policy will need to respond to these broader influences. For example, if global warming, land degradation and other environmental factors further increase the numbers of 'environmental refugees', special forms of educational provision will become necessary. Unlike with normal refugees, the possibility of these people returning to uninhabitable land is remote.

There are also environmental impacts at a classroom level. Teachers in some London schools now regularly listen to the weather/pollution forecast in the morning because this will determine how they teach. In a class where 20 per cent of children suffer pollution-related asthma, the general level of concentration is considerably less when air quality is bad. In Seaford, Sussex, a special school, Pilgrims, opened in 1994 specifically to cater for children suffering from asthma. The cost per pupil is £21,000 each year. This form of provision is unlikely to become available on the required scale, so the response to asthma will need to pervade all schools.

In Mexico City, it is now recognized that school attendance is poor on the days when the air quality is poor. In the winter, schools start later to avoid the worst pollution in the early morning. In the Bronx, children sometimes cannot go outside at playtime because of air pollution, with resultant behaviour difficulties. Will schools generally become more flexible to accommodate these problems?

In northern Bohemia, 40,000 smog masks were issued to schoolchildren in 1990 because the incidence of pollution-related illness was so high. In the UK, some schoolchildren have been issued with special sun hats to protect them from ultraviolet radiation, and in New Zealand hats and 'cover-up' clothing are a mandatory part of school uniform. In these circumstances schools must do more than give out the means of protection, they must educate as to the importance of protection – which of course distracts from other curriculum needs.

Direct prevention is another aspect. The effects of alcohol abuse by pregnant women on the brains of their unborn children are most serious during the first three weeks of pregnancy. Health care intervention is therefore too late, so education at school is the only route to addressing this problem. Personal safety lessons will eventually need to go beyond 'Don't talk to strangers' and reflect local environmental hazards. Those living near a chemical plant should learn that in the event of a toxic release they should run against the wind. Although counter-intuitive, this gets you away from the exposure more quickly. This is not science fiction. Children living in Bhopal now learn this strategy as a part of their cultural tradition.

The relationship between environmental change and education is usually only evident in the form of environmental education, which gives an impression that the problem is distant and 'out there'. Soon schools will need to recognize the effects of environmental change on their day-to-day running – the problem is 'right here', and that is an uncomfortable admission for governments, which will inevitably mean delays in adopting necessary strategies.

Children who experience environmental problems may also experience psycho-social problems. In regions where children suffer directly from environmental victimization, involvement in resisting that victimization can be both constructive and therapeutic. Sharon Stephens reports on the work of the Viola environmental group in the Bryansk region of south-west Russia, which suffers from Chernobyl fallout and industrial toxins. Between 1986 and 1990 parents and teachers had noticed a sharp increase in depression, passivity and aggression among young people:

> This situation improved markedly, as children (some as young as 10 years old) became involved in monitoring local pollution – drawing up maps of the effects of acid rain and measuring levels of chemical and radioactive contamination.
>
> One group of children found high levels of mercury in ponds and ditches where they played. They traced the chemical to a local factory producing mercury vapour lamps for the military. The children, together with Viola members and some parents and teachers, then made formal protests to local authorities and factory officials. This resulted in the factory installing clean-up equipment . . . Another group of children located radioactive hot spots on local playgrounds. Sand on the playgrounds was removed and the play area paved over with asphalt, minimizing dangers from direct contact with radioactive soil.[11]

This form of educative response is a striking contrast to the probable reaction to aggression among children in schools in, say, London, some of whose behaviour problems may also stem from environmental exposure to heavy metals. The difference is that the Russian child is accorded the status of an environmental victim who suffers a health problem, because the cause is so apparent. The schoolchildren in London are not, and so are just nuisances to be punished.

The Russian example raises the most significant area for change, which is not in curriculum, pedagogy or diets. It concerns teacher attitudes. When children are given the label 'special needs', 'learning disabilities' or 'victims', teachers are sympathetic, and dealing appropriately with related behaviour and achievement problems becomes a matter of professional pride. Without the labels, this rarely happens. A teacher in a New York school for children who suffer intellectual and behaviour problems because their mothers used crack while they were pregnant presents her outlook in a constructive manner: 'They are going to be very violent and disturbed people unless they are taught a different pattern of behaviour.'[12] But would she have made such a positive comment had she met the same children in a mainstream school, and was not directly aware of the reason for their behaviour?

Those children just one notch above the cut-off point for the special needs labels are usually seen as disruptive, deviant and discipline problems – and the response is to punish. The cut-off point varies widely between and within countries, and even within schools. It usually reflects the cash available to support children with special needs, not an objective identification of those needs.

The result is that children who would be seen as disabled in one school are seen as deviant in another. Teachers treat clinical problems as discipline problems, and the resultant punitive ethos ends up constructing a degenerative spiral of injustice and resistance, which must eventually contribute to the increasing numbers of disaffected youth and marginalized adults.

In many settings punishment goes well beyond a reprimand. In Southern Africa it is not unusual for children to be hospitalized following corporal punishment by teachers. In Zimbabwe a 7-year-old child died after he was beaten by his mathematics teacher for giving a wrong answer to a question. In the context of environmental causation, most unjust are the punishment regimes in special schools for children with behaviour problems. One unpublished government report reveals how children supposedly 'in care' were 'regularly kicked, punched, thrown, kneed and viciously beaten . . . In one case two boys were whipped from head to toe . . . [Others were] punched in the stomach and then kicked across the room.' This is not in an impoverished, backward nation – it happened in Britain.[13]

Another related spiral of injustice is even less conspicuous. Environmental chemicals may well be a cause or a contributing factor among schoolchildren whose behaviour is seen as difficult or who are diagnosed as suffering attention deficit hyperactivity disorder. In the rich nations these children may well be treated with a drug such as Ritalin. In the USA,

Ritalin use is ten times greater than in France or Britain: 1.3 million children take it daily. Such drugs may control the immediate problem, but they might also depress general intellectual functioning – another iatrogenic effect. The children suffer a double blow to their intellectual potential, which would not happen if the original environmental impact were avoided.

Even if science were eventually to conclude that there is only a minimal link between environmental chemicals and school problems, little harm would be done by teachers adopting a more positive approach to problematic pupils – a socio-environmental 'precautionary principle'. To overestimate the link between environmental chemicals and school problems would simply lead to teachers treating more pupils with greater respect, and adopting more constructive approaches to their difficulties. To underestimate the link means that teachers will punish pupils who are seen as deviant, when they should be supporting pupils who in reality have a disability.

## Achieving change

As agents of change, campaign groups such as CLEAR (Campaign for Lead-free Air) in the UK have had a significant influence.[14] Laws have been made, regulations enforced, public awareness increased and health responses improved. But still only half the cars in the UK use unleaded petrol. Although effective in the short term, activism can have little long-term impact unless governments are convinced of the need for change. Paradoxically, fundamental improvement may become greater in the poorer countries where the problems are more obvious. During the elections for city governor in Bangkok in 1996, Bhichit Rattakud stood on the basis of making petrol lead-free. His supporters sprayed themselves with grey metallic paint and canvassed as the 'lead men'. For a politician to think that he can get elected on an anti-lead ticket is a remarkable innovation in local politics, indicating the perceived degree of public concern.

Local activists achieve change through short-term, well-targeted campaigns. One German group tracked the manufacture of a solvent glue, commonly used by street children in Brazil, to a German factory. Activists identified the neurotoxic solvent and persuaded the company to replace this chemical with one that was less harmful. In the Netherlands, where the national disability day is marked by wearing a flower, environmental groups have pointed out the irony. The flowers probably result from exploitative child labour and exposure to pesticides in poorer nations – which causes disability.

On the level of personal change, there are reports that some individuals are taking drastic action to avoid perceived environmental threats. In Brownsville, Texas, where pollution blowing across the border from the

Mexican *maquiladoras* factories is seen as causing severe birth impairments, some young couples are moving away from the area before they start a family. Scientifically this might not be a rational response, but as an indication of the social perception of a problem, the behaviour is significant. Will we eventually see clean countries promoting themselves as breeding grounds for the rich? New Zealand, for example, would be an obvious location for those who originate from the polluted cities of southern China and Taiwan, and there are signs that this is already happening.

The use of new technology to prevent toxins entering the environment provides another aspect. The concept of 'closed systems' is rapidly gaining ground. These not only prevent public poisoning but also save industries considerable sums because valuable materials are not then lost through the factory chimney. Local environmental NGOs, such as the Good Neighbor Project in the USA, work with local industries to minimize risk through, for example, making the throughput of hazardous chemicals more efficient and therefore reducing the amount that is stored.[15] Technical strategies do not have to be high-tech. An initiative among the Amazon gold miners uses two very simple devices to prevent the loss of mercury into the air and into the river, which can be made from scrap metal or local wood at a cost of about $30 each, a sum that can be recovered in one day.[16]

International and national mobilization has been most impressive in relation to *absence*-EMID, principally iodine deficiency. The International Council for the Control of Iodine Deficiency Disorders now facilitates significant action at national levels – the mandatory iodization of salt, for example. Research centres such as the Program against Micronutrient Malnutrition at Emory University, Atlanta, take a broader view in relation to a range of 'hidden hunger' problems. Local NGOs are usually well networked through UNICEF or WHO, and are able to get at the 'devil in the detail' of national strategies. A UNICEF report from the Gorakhpur Environmental Action Group, in India, highlights the problem caused by iodine being washed from salt transported in open railway wagons. There can be a delay of between 6 and 12 months waiting for closed wagons, and wagons used to carry fertilizers and pesticides are sometimes then used to carry salt without cleaning.[17]

Results are becoming tangible. In India the ID Programme has reduced iodine-related intellectual decline from 92 to 11 per 1000 in some regions. There are also signs of success in relation to other micro-nutrients. Iron supplements for anaemic children in India and West Java are shown to have improved their IQ, memory and perception. A project in Guatemala run by the Institute of Nutrition of Central America, which provides a high-protein supplement called Atole to young children, has demonstrated that this can counteract the forms of intellectual decline usually associated with poverty. But from another perspective, this provides yet further evidence that poor nutrition and poverty in infancy can undermine the benefits of schooling.[18]

It is interesting to compare explanations as to why government responses have been most tangible in relation to lead and iodine. Lansdown and Yule propose five reasons which, operating simultaneously, inspired action in relation to lead:

- growth of consumerism and ecological awareness;

- the dangers of high-level exposure having been well established, it was easier to argue the threat from low levels;

- children were seen as prime victims and this had an emotional appeal;

- the problem of lead in petrol has a reasonably simple technical solution that was politically acceptable;

- the topic provided good editorial copy.[19]

Basil Hetzel identifies comparable factors in relation to iodine:

- the problem was of sufficient magnitude to justify a major allocation of resources;

- there were effective preventive measures suitable for use on a mass scale;

- there was an available delivery system;

- there were practical methods for monitoring and surveillance of the programme so that it could be shown to be effective.[20]

If these explanations are compared with those relating to other environ-mental movements, one aspect is absent – the participation and activism of those who suffer. For obvious reasons, achieving change to reduce EMID is almost wholly dependent on social action *on behalf of others*. Because this can appear paternalistic, and charity is not now an acceptable approach to human problems, EMID could well be sidelined through the desire to comply with fashion.

More broadly, iodine and lead are simple single-substance issues – they present identifiable targets with a tidy campaign profile. But EMID is caused by a myriad of factors in addition to lead and iodine deficiency. Multifaceted problems are conceptually messy and difficult to fit into simple sound bites, so they are much harder to change. It is only governments and the major international agencies that have the capacity to attack untidy problems on the required scale.

It would be easy to finish *Terminus Brain* at this point on a note of optimism, suggesting that communities can, with a little adjustment, respond adequately to the problems posed by EMID. Science can find a cure for the problems it causes, and social systems can adapt.

But even if the cures could be made available equitably on the required scale, which is improbable, do we really want to create a world of detox schools and mandatory toxin testing, in which an annual trip to the health farm is a normal part of a child's upbringing? Environmental activism may be therapeutic for children, but it is intrinsically conflictual and will not contribute to sustainable society in countries that already have seemingly intractable social divides. The cures are not cures – they are just more symptoms of the ill.

---

## Notes

1. John Elkington, *The Poisoned Womb* (Penguin: Harmondsworth, 1985), pp. 45, 236.

2. 'Ayurveda drugs can cure metal toxicity', *Sunday Times of India*, 24 December 1995, p. 5.

3. Alexander Dorozynski, 'Paris finds high lead concentrations in its poorer children', *British Medical Journal* (1993), **307**, 523.

4. C.B. Travis *et al.*, *Environmental Toxins: Psychological, Behavioral, and Sociocultural Aspects* (American Psychological Association: Washington, DC, 1989).

5. H.L. Needleman *et al.*, 'Deficits in psychologic and classroom performance of children with elevated dentine lead levels', *New England Journal of Medicine* (1979), **300**, 689–95.

6. R. Lansdown *et al.*, 'Relationships between blood-lead, intelligence, attainment and behaviour in school children', in M. Rutter and R. Jones (eds), *Lead versus Health* (Wiley & Sons: London, 1982).

7. Herbert L. Needleman *et al.*, 'The long-term effects of exposure to low doses of lead in childhood: an 11-year follow-up report', *New England Journal of Medicine* (1990), **322**(2), 83–8.

8. Theo Colborn, *Our Stolen Future* (Little, Brown & Co.: London, 1996), p. 235.

9. Basil S. Hetzel, *The Story of Iodine Deficiency* (Oxford University Press: Oxford, 1989), p. 90.

10. J. Larry Brown and Ernesto Pollitt, 'Malnutrition, poverty and intellectual development', *Scientific American* (1996), **274**(2), 26–31.

11. Sharon Stephens, 'Reflections on environmental justice: children as victims and actors', *Social Justice* (1996), **23**(4), 62–86.

12. Geordie Greig, '"Crack kids" give America a new lesson', *Sunday Times*, 8 March 1992, p. 21.

13. Roger Dobson, '25-year cover-up of victims in care', *Independent*, 20 June 1996, p. 7.

14. Des Wilson, *The Lead Scandal: The Fight to Save Children from Damage by Lead in Petrol* (Heinemann: London, 1983).

15. Sanford Lewis and Diane Henkels, 'Good neighbor agreements: a tool for environmental and social justice', *Social Justice* (1996), **23**(4), 134–51.

16. Andy Coghan, 'Midas touch could end Amazon's pollution', *New Scientist* (1995), **196**, 10.

17. UNICEF, *Iodine Deficiency in Trans Saryu Plains* (Gorakhpur Environmental Action Group: Gorakhpur, 1993), pp. 26–32.

18. Brown and Pollitt, *op. cit.* (n. 10), p. 28.

19. R. Lansdown and W. Yule, *Lead Toxicity: History and Environmental Impact* (Johns Hopkins University Press: Baltimore, 1986), p. 271.

20. Hetzel, *op. cit.* (n. 9), p. 148.

# PART IV

# The Ecological Environment

# CHAPTER 9

# The Brain in the Ecosystem

*[The] substance of humans and their environment is wholly chemically based . . . humans represent organized islands of chemicals set within an ocean of foreign chemicals.*[1]

The brain survives not only in relation to its mobile bodily environment and the social environment that we create, but also within the ecosystem – 'an ocean of foreign chemicals'. Human existence is increasingly perceived as part of the ecosystem, but the place of the human brain as a distinct eco-entity has received very little attention outside evolutionary perspectives.

We need to be aware of the broad relationships between the natural ecosystem, human-made environmental change and the threat to the brain as an organism. There is relatively little empirical research in this field, so an awareness of the knowledge gaps is crucial. More broadly, we need to consider that the brain has evolved progressively over millions of years because of a positive interaction between it and its environment. We are now in a new era – it seems that for the first time in human evolution this interaction can culminate in adverse consequences for the brain, and even the possibility of regressive brain evolution.

## Natural hazards

The basis of *Terminus Brain* is so-called 'environmental change' – but change from what? It would be wrong to assume that the natural world represented an eco-idyll, which intrinsically accommodated the human brain, posing no hazards. A clearer idea of what is meant by the natural state, and how this could have an adverse impact on human intellectual resources without the radical dynamics of modernity, underpins the broader ecological perspective.

The natural *presence* of potential hazards is tangible in relation to heavy metals, which occur in most soils. In trace amounts these are essential for plant, animal and human growth. Between 2700 and 6000 tonnes of mercury are released naturally from the earth's crust each year, for example.

**157**

Occasionally, natural levels of heavy metals in a locality are very high, as in the region of the submarine volcanoes in the eastern Mediterranean. We seem to know nothing about how natural hazards such as these might have adversely affected the intellectual resources of specific communities.

There is a little evidence about the impact of natural radiation. In regions of Yangjiang County, Guangdong Province, China, where environmental gamma radiation is about three times higher than the norm, the frequency of Down's syndrome is reported to be 'significantly higher' than among similar communities elsewhere.[2] Similarly, in a coastal region of Kerala, India, where the radiation comes from a thorium-containing monazite mineral in the soil, a significant increase in Down's syndrome and severe mental retardation has been documented over a number of years.[3]

The Indian example immediately brings up the common omission in the perception of the natural state of things – the human eco-actors. The threat from radiation in Kerala may be fundamentally non-human, but the problem has certainly been exacerbated by human behaviour. In many places the sea sand containing the thorium has been moved from a natural location and dumped by a mining company, Indian Rare Earths Ltd, to prevent houses from collapsing as a result of its mining activities.

Interestingly in the China case, although the brain was affected, cancer and other congenital defects showed no increase. This might suggest that there are forms of biological adaptation to the high-radiation environment among populations which live and evolve in such regions, but that these adaptations do not operate so effectively in relation to the brain. But as yet there are no empirical conclusions.

It is also now proposed that the effect of human-made radioactive substances on cells seems to be different from, and perhaps more dangerous than, the impact of natural radiation. Chris Busby's 'second event theory' suggests that, from a human-made exposure, a cell can be damaged twice within a critical period of ten hours. The second event disables vital DNA repair mechanisms triggered by the first. This sequence is highly unlikely in relation to natural background radiation.[4]

The importance of the difference between potential threats in their natural or human-made forms is only just coming to the attention of scientists. Lead is a central example because when emitted as a petrol additive it is not in its basic mineral form; nor is it in the form in which it is used for most animal experiments. Research into the differing effects of human-made and natural hazards may well eventually challenge standard arguments from polluters that an impact on human well-being is not hazardous because it is lower than natural levels of exposure.

Natural *absence*-EMID has been documented for centuries in Europe and China, in relation to iodine. In 1848, King Carlo Alberto of Sardinia commissioned a study finding 120,000 cretins and idiots, whose condition was caused by iodine deficiency, among a population of about 36 million in France. But while we know of the existence of iodine disorders from a medical perspective, less has been recorded about the social impact. What little mention there is tends to imply acceptance rather than any recognition of a social problem. In twentieth-century Europe preventive measures, although not completely adequate, have combated widespread iodine-related intellectual decline. Had this not happened, Europe's intellectual resources would now be significantly different. In Germany, Italy, Spain, Portugal, Romania, Greece and Turkey there is still cause for concern.[5]

Within pre-industrial communities, general nutritional levels must have been sufficient to permit adequate intellectual functioning, or populations would not have survived. Adequate nutrition was more a clear-cut matter of life or death. The difference now is that we have evolved ways to feed the global population which prevent death, but often the nature of the food is such that it does not permit optimum intellectual development. The Green Revolution has a significant impact by decreasing the nutritional value of the basic diet for millions of people.

The most worrying aspect of *absence*-EMID is the scale of our ignorance. In the wake of current biodiversity losses, are we sure that we are not going to lose environmental agents that are crucial for the functioning of the brain, but are not yet identified in this role? We have only recently become aware of the importance of iron for optimum intellectual functioning. And iron is a simple, common element. There is one certainty: the human brain evolved to its present condition through biological interaction within the rich biodiversity as it existed a few decades ago, and this situation is changing fast.

The clinical awareness of biological *synergism* in the body (Chapter 3) raises an important question. How significant are similar patterns in the ecosystem? If natural minerals have been washed from the soil, are the soil and plant life more likely to take up toxic human-made substitutes? Artificial nitrogenous fertilizers change the pH level of soil, which affects the uptake of heavy metals by plants. The presence of environmental toxins such as thiocyanates reduces the uptake of iodine by vegetables such as cabbage and ladies' fingers, thus creating the absence problem in human diet.[6] Dr Vandana Shiva, director of the Research Institute for Natural Policy, India, points out that the over-use of NPK (nitrogen, phosphorus and potassium) fertilizers leads to micro-nutrient deficiencies of zinc, iron, copper and magnesium. There is a growing awareness of eco-synergism, but no comprehensive conclusions in relation to eco-synergism and EMID.

There is one further area of ignorance: very little is known about how EMID affects wild animals. There is research about the levels of agents such as heavy metals in farm animals, and we know a great deal about neurotoxins and the brains of laboratory animals. There is even anecdotal evidence that iodine deficiency affects domestic animals, such as dogs.[7]

But it is only recently that researchers have considered effects of environmental chemicals on wild animals' migratory behaviour, their ability to hunt or sense danger, nest-building, rearing of young and other survival skills.[8] Even from this it is not clear to what degree animal intelligence, as opposed to instinct, has been affected.

Even the most basic of organisms can be considered to display forms of intelligence, as outlined in the next chapter. If other living creatures or simple organisms suffer a decline in their basic intelligence, what impact might this have on the overall ecosystem, and ultimately on us?

## Ecological mechanisms

Beyond the basic state of environmental agents, we need also to be aware of mechanisms within the ecosystem that change and route those agents. Three of the key mechanisms are

- *Reconcentration*: the accumulation of a substance that has been dissolved or dissipated in air, soil or water, much as a tea strainer reconcentrates tea leaves.

- *Conversion*: a change in a chemical, which may present it in a form more hazardous to humans or in a form that is vital for human life.

- *Vectoring*: the routeing and carrying of environmental agents (or health hazards) from one place to another. Vectors have both magnitude and direction; for example, rivers, winds or insects.

The *reconcentration* mechanism is well known in relation to fish and shellfish. And, as common sense would suggest, fish-eating fish such as tuna reconcentrate toxins to an even greater degree. The levels of mercury in predatory fish can be 10,000 to 1,000,000 times the concentrations in the surrounding water.[9] If we did not eat fish, they would probably be classed as an ecological mechanism defending, not posing a threat to, the human brain.

Reconcentration is not restricted to animals. Reed beds have much the same effect. Vegetables and fruit also reconcentrate toxins, and it is the exact location of the toxins that can be important. Organophosphates accumulate in the skin of carrots. So too do the essential micro-nutrients. Therefore skinning the vegetable might solve the *presence* problem but may contribute to an *absence* one. But reconcentration does not always lead to environmental hazards. As explained later, the reconcentration of iodine in a seaweed, kelp, is essential to make that micro-nutrient available to humans.

Rain too plays its part. Acid rain appears to be a significant explanation for excess mercury in the aquatic environment.[10] So-called 'background' radiation may be relatively harmless while dissipated in the atmosphere, but heavy rain brings it to earth in reconcentrated amounts. (This phenomenon was a factor in the empirical evidence about radiation EMID in Chapter 6.) Commercial discourse, especially from the nuclear industry, promotes the term 'background', which from another viewpoint is synonymous with 'ineluctable' – present everywhere, so there is no escape.

*Conversion* was central to the story of mercury poisoning by the Chisso plant at Minamata Bay, Japan, in the 1950s and 1960s. Around 30 tonnes of *inorganic* mercury were discharged into the bay, and this was considered safe because mercury was thought to be relatively harmless to humans in this form. But inorganic mercury is converted into the *organic* form (methylmercury) by micro-organisms in sediments, and is then taken up and reconcentrated by fish and shellfish. Humans around Minamata Bay ate the fish containing mercury in an organic form, which is quickly harmful to the brain, causing permanent damage. At the time the discharges into the bay were made, this practice was thought to be safe because science did not understand the conversion mechanism.

The importance of understanding conversion mechanisms in relation to non-living biomass is demonstrated in a letter to *Nature* in 1994.[11] The high level of mercury in the blood of fish-eating people in the Amazon is usually attributed to pollution from the conspicuous source, gold mining. But high mercury levels have been noted in fish up to 250 kilometres away from the mining area, which raised a question about other sources of mercury pollution. The mystery was that there were no obvious industrial sources. In these regions, deforestation is happening on a large scale, and fires are part of the process. Mercury occurs naturally in biomass and, under natural circumstances, the release is controlled. But burning trees and vegetation suddenly releases this mercury, leaving it loosely bound to the ash, from which it quickly gets washed into water sources. The authors of the letter proposed that fires accompanying deforestation may be a source of mercury in fish of equal significance to the more obvious mining activities.

Again, conversion mechanisms are not intrinsically hazardous. They also change environmental agents into forms of micro-nutrients that are available and necessary for human development.

The possible effects of global warming demonstrate the need to understand *vectors*. In *Planetary Overload*, A. J. McMichael predicts that increased temperature and resultant rainfall in Australia would permit vector-borne diseases to extend to higher latitudes or higher altitudes, because of the increase in surface water. New rivers and lakes would create the vectors for mosquitoes (themselves technically vectors), and these could spread south bringing arboviral infections such as Murray Valley encephalitis, which can impair the brain.

Tick-borne infectious diseases such as Lyme disease, which causes residual brain damage, may spread further in the USA if the climate alters.[12] Changes in land cover may create new problems. There is concern in that the spread of bracken, a green fern, may pose a hazard because it harbours the Lyme disease tick.

Gravity is usually not acknowledged as representing a vector, yet it is probably the most significant. Gravity dictates that naturally occurring micro-nutrients seep from high land to low; so too do water-vectored toxins. High-lying regions then threaten the brain through *absence*-EMID; low-lying regions through *presence*-EMID. Eventually both top and bottom of our habitat become inhospitable for the brain, and this coincides with an increasing need for habitable land because of population growth.

Most significantly, the vital environmental nutrients end up in the same place as the poisons. Nothing is known about the synergistic effects between the poisons and the micro-nutrients when they gravitate together in low-lying parts of the ecosystem, which perhaps could render the micro-nutrients unavailable to the ecological cycle in a form eventually useful to the brain.

Like the other eco-mechanisms, vectors of course serve favourable functions as well. They take away concentrations of naturally occurring hazardous substances. They provide the routes along which the vital micro-nutrients become available to humans.

James Lovelock provides a broad view of eco-mechanisms in relation to *absence*-EMID, seamlessly linking the bodily and ecological environments – embracing conversion, reconcentration and vectors – and then the possible human precipitant of an environmentally mediated threat:

> The thyroid gland . . . harvests the meagre supplies of iodine from the internal bodily environment and converts them into iodine-bearing hormones which regulate our metabolism . . . Certain large marine algae, laminaria, may perform a similar function to the thyroid gland but on a planetary scale. These long straps of seaweed . . . concentrate the element iodine from sea-water and process from their harvest a curious set of iodine-bearing substances . . . One way or another the iodine of the sea, concentrated by laminaria, is blown through the air to land surfaces of the earth and is absorbed by mammals like ourselves . . . The algae which perform this vital function exist along a thin line surrounding the continents and islands of the world . . .

> *When I hear that there are proposals for the large-scale farming of kelp,*
> *which is the common name for laminaria, I find the prospect more disturbing*
> *than the effects of any of the industrial hazards . . . The breeding of strains*
> *of kelp which gave better yields of alginate would be an early step in farming*
> *practice. Such strains might lose their capacity to harvest iodine from the sea.*[13]

Like so much of the necessary knowledge, the basic facts wound together
by Lovelock are not new. It has been known for centuries that communities which live near the sea are unlikely to suffer iodine deficiency. The
Chinese Emperor Shen-Nung (*c.* 2737 BC) wrote of the seaweed sargasso
as a remedy for iodine-related disorders, and the idea comes up again in
the writings of Ge-Khun (between AD 317 and 419) and persists throughout history.[14]

The biological eco-mechanisms are therefore neutral, but generally
favourable to human existence. They constitute natural defences against
neurotoxins, and they make and distribute the micro-nutrients in forms
available to the human body. Despite the potential hazards of the geological
world, the eco-mechanisms have for millions of years created a general
environment that is conducive to the existence of the human brain. If it
were otherwise, we would not have our present intellectual ability – a
thought we should keep in mind when regulating the impact of human
behaviour on the natural state of things. Why, for example, when it is
known that the natural level of lead in dust is about 15 parts per million,
does the UK Department of the Environment set a 'safe level' for the
current human-made environment of the human brain of 2000?

## Environmental change

So what is different – what is the difference between the natural
environment and the result of human-made environmental change?
Environmental change stems from human behaviour that falls under the
broad heading of modernity. Social theorists provide detailed elaborations,
but there are three basic dynamics that can underpin a general
understanding: things are now *bigger*, *faster* and *more mixed up*.

## Bigger, faster . . .

We now have lead in polar ice, and PCBs in polar bears. There is certainly
something very different about the scale of human-made environmental
change. Ice samples in Greenland reveal that there has been a 20-fold
increase in lead pollution since the industrial revolution. As a result,
according to Dr Clair Patterson, most humans now have body burdens
of lead 500 to 1000 times greater than their prehistoric ancestors.[15] The
totality of human exposure to chemicals such as DDT and the synthetic

hormone-disrupting chemicals is something completely new. As described in Chapter 6, the totality of the Green Revolution fuels the *absence*-EMID threat. Global warming could have an impact. Acute high temperatures can adversely affect early foetal development,[16] cerebral malaria may become more widespread and a decline in the nutritional value of food might affect new regions.

Just the scale of human activities can create environmental hazards that threaten the brain. Human-made chemicals are not the sole cause of *presence*-EMID. Hazards can arise because the eco-mechanisms that might otherwise render natural toxins harmless are defeated by human activity. The creation of reservoirs at the La Grande complex in Canada provides an example. The resultant flooding of woodland caused a rapid increase in decaying vegetation. Vegetation converts naturally occurring inorganic mercury into the hazardous organic form. If remaining in the vegetation, this would eventually evaporate safely. But the increase in water not only precipitated this rapid, large-scale biological *conversion*, it also created a *vector* permitting the organic mercury to be taken up by fish, which then *reconcentrated* it. Fish at La Grande were found to have levels of methyl-mercury five times higher than those in fish in nearby freshwater lakes. While the ecological chain of events was itself natural and unproblematic, the size and speed of the human-made precipitant turned a potential hazard into an actual one.

The most significant aspect of scale is, of course, exponential population growth, which results from and drives the dynamics of modernity. Projections propose that the global population may increase by between 50 and 100 per cent in the next forty or fifty years. This means that in four decades we will need to create homes, food, infrastructure and energy sources on a scale that more or less equals what exists now; and to do this while reducing environmental impacts that could impair the intellectual potential of this new mass of humanity.

### . . . and more mixed up

The most significant aspect of human *mixing up* stems from the ability, since the middle of the nineteenth century, to produce synthetic chemicals – we learned to create new chemicals from simple, naturally occurring chemicals. Dioxin is a pertinent example. There are now over 3.4 million known chemicals, and in excess of 5000 new ones are introduced for industrial use every year.

The case of cerebral malaria, which if it does not kill often creates a mental impairment, provides one example of the broader mix-up of the modernity dynamics. Mosquitoes and parasites are fast becoming resistant to insecticides because of the over-use of these synthetic chemicals, which increases the disease vector. The infection is also becoming drug-resistant because of the massive scale of the use of insecticides and curative drugs. Some of the drugs themselves can impair the brain – an iatrogenic effect (Chapter 6). A recent awareness of genetic vulnerability will provide another dimension (Chapters 3 and 4). According to Dr Bill McGuire of the Institute of Molecular Medicine in Oxford, it seems that children in The Gambia are seven times more likely to die or suffer brain damage from malaria because they produce a high level of a hormone called tumour necrosis factor.

To this chemical soup can be added another social dimension, dam-building. Dams create vast new areas of still water. This not only increases the mosquito population, but also leads to a further increase in the scale of pesticides and drugs use. An escalation of malaria and Japanese encephalitis is predicted in connection with the Narmada dam in India. A proposed dam in Malaysia will flood an area the size of Singapore – the biggest, fastest human-made flooding in history. The increase in surface water owing to global warming may further drive the problem. The sudden appearance of a predominantly rural problem, cerebral malaria, in urban regions of India in 1996 foreshadows new 'mix-up' consequences of new 'mix-up' environmental change.

The paradox arising from the relentless modernity mix-up is that some forms of hazardous human-made change may now *mitigate* the adverse effects of other forms of harmful activity. In the Rhine basin area, heavy metal pollution was a major problem in the mid- to late 1960s. Emissions to the air and surface water have since fallen, but soil pollution has not improved because soil retains the substances longer. At the same time, the pH level of agricultural land has been maintained at an unnaturally high level by the application of lime, and this reduces the capacity of soils to vector heavy metals. Even small declines in the soil's pH may lead to a significant increase in crop uptake of heavy metals.

The situation now, according to research funded by the Netherlands government, is that 'the consistent liming of agricultural soils, particularly near industrialized regions with high cumulative inputs of heavy metals and acid deposition, becomes increasingly important in order to control sharp and sudden increases in the uptake of trace metals by crops'.[17] *Decreasing* the use of artificial fertilizers and the accompanying environmental hazards may *increase* the heavy metal threat to humans. Current EU policy is encouraging a reduction in agricultural land usage, with farmland reverting to 'natural' forests, and this could speed up the leaching of heavy metals from the soil into drinking water supplies.

The alarming part of the modernity mix-up is that we end up with lock-in situations such as this. We then have to view human products such as factories and fertilizers as having a significant potential for ecological interaction in their own right, and that is an uncomfortable conceptualization for many ecologists. Human intervention is on such a scale that there is now virtually no such thing as a totally natural ecosystem.

Causal chains can therefore appear very complex, and this complexity leads to a significant misconception about human-made environmental hazards. We view human intervention as a mechanism that *dissipates* hazardous substances from nodal points: mercury from waste pipes into rivers, PCBs from factory chimneys into the air, CFCs from aerosols and fridges into the ozone layer.

This is correct analysis, but it can be a misleading way to envision the problem – dissipation is only one small stage in the overall process. In the context of the whole ecosystem, the threat posed to human well-being by environmental change is better conceived as *vectoring*. Modernity creates new super-vectors from the potential threats posed by the geological world to the human body.

The vision of *presence*-EMID should be of a modernity super-vector from environmental agents in their elemental form, such as mercury or uranium, direct to the human brain: a new superhighway, which by-passes the natural defences provided by the biological eco-mechanisms. The same image can be drawn in relation to *absence*-EMID. Modernity constructs a super-vector from the geological world of no micro-nutrients, to the human brain, by-passing the vital biological eco-mechanisms that create the nutrients in forms that our body can assimilate. The cliché that humans are becoming 'more distanced from the natural world' is misleading. True, we are becoming more distanced from those crucial eco-mechanisms, but the modernity super-vectors bring us dangerously *closer* to the unfavourable environment of the geological world.

These super-vectors are very evident in environmental health problems. The spread of disease through increased human mobility, the trade in foodstuffs and plants, and the mass availability of narcotic drugs thousands of miles from their natural source are all obvious examples. The dynamics of cerebral malaria (described above) can be seen as modernity creating a new super-vector from a relatively localized and controllable disease, direct to the brains of far greater numbers of the global population.

It seems no coincidence that the aim of commerce is to get raw materials from their place of origin, often the geological world, to consumers, in the form of manufactured products, by the shortest possible line. The development of commercial activity has many benefits, but it also constructs modernity super-vectors which carry along with them the hazards that we call 'environmental change'.

## The evolutionary context

The other perspective on the brain in an ecosystem comes from the evolutionary theorists. But discussion of the current environmental threat to human intelligence has not yet been framed in the light of this body of knowledge. And the evolutionary thinkers rarely extend their understanding about the past to inform the present about the possible future. Our knowledge of our history should be a major survival skill, but in relation to the brain this is not yet so.

Much has been written addressing the question of how, over millions of years, the human brain evolved progressively in the context of its environment. Yet by comparison little has been written about how, also in the context of its environment, we might ensure that the human brain we now possess does not decline from its current favourable form. Future historians may view this as a strange bias – if history still exists. From the perspective of human survival, the bias is akin to driving a car around while looking out of the back window. We do not need extensive abstract futurology, just to look where we're going in the light of where we've come from.

The bias appears even more curious when we remember how problematic it is to assess intelligence from archaeological records. We can only make a guess based on our increasing brain size and the apparent progression of human achievement, so conclusions are highly speculative. As Thomas Wynn, one of the theorists in this area, concludes, 'we cannot give Neanderthals the Stanford–Binet' IQ test.[18] By contrast, we do have empirical, although imperfect, means to assess intelligence in current and future populations.

In *The Runaway Brain*, Christopher Wills provides a very plausible explanation of the evolutionary 'loop' that has probably conditioned the human brain into its present form. Throughout human evolution the amount of brain development that happens after birth has slowly but constantly increased, far beyond that of other species. Consequently, he argues, the degree to which our brain is shaped by the external environment has also increased.

Wills elaborates: 'Such selective pressures would have been very different from those that shaped our teeth, or our pelvis, for they were in the form of *intellectual* rather than physical challenges.' Speech, tools, fire, clothing and shelter were the product of the evolving brain, but these also then constituted the environment that posed the challenges for the brain, leading to further evolution. We harnessed fire, and then had to develop the intellectual abilities to stop us getting our fingers burned. Wills concludes: 'If this feedback loop is real, it does much to explain why our own evolution has been so clearly different from that of other organisms.'[19]

And to this vision of a feedback loop must be added the role of the environmental chemical soup which was broadly favourable to the brain's organic development.

But is the prognosis for the brain forever onward and upward? No, according to current evolutionary theory; the biological development of the human brain has reached a pinnacle, irrespective of EMID.[20] Positive genetic evolution required small populations (peripheral isolates), which were cut off from their parent species so that progressive genetic changes were preserved and perpetuated. These populations then survived better and eventually outlived their static progenitors. Modernity dictates that such populations are unlikely to exist in the future, so this mechanism for genetic progression has virtually disappeared.

This stabilizing dynamic is compounded by our benevolent morality, which (in theory) makes welfare and health care broadly available irrespective of the genetic potential of individuals. The survival of the fittest is not now an acceptable ethos, and therefore the self-selective breeding of the most intelligent cadres is no longer a route to progressive brain evolution.

If the human brain has reached a biological plateau, might EMID precipitate a descent that is, in the very long term, inevitable? Indicators are masked in two ways. First, we already perceive a massive variation in the abilities of the contemporary human brain, even without any biological differences, so any biological regression would be hard to detect. Second, because significant evolution of the brain takes millions of years, it is probably too soon to identify any regressive effect caused by environmental change in the manner that we can identify the progressive evolution of the brain throughout human history.

But despite this masking of change, the debate about the evolution and uniqueness of human intelligence might soon embrace a new realization of our age: *our brain could now pose a threat to its own positive evolution through its adverse interaction with its environment.* And it does this knowingly. Choosing to expose populations to lead through car use is not akin to a monkey that injures its brain because it falls out of a tree. There is little that is accidental about our current relationship with our environment.

Have we reached an era in which the scale and nature of the threats are such that our brain has already entered a degenerative spiral? We do not know. But in theory it might be argued that current EMID *could* be a precursor of regressive brain evolution in specific populations, if sufficient numbers in those populations were affected. We could perhaps now make the evolutionary 'loop' spin backwards.

There could be a natural selection 'trade-off'. We seem to have evolved bigger brains at the cost of a smaller digestive system, which therefore requires high-quality food.[21] If food supplies become poor-quality or contaminated, this might eventually favour the selection of humans with a bigger gut but a resultantly smaller brain. New research also challenges the established belief that environmental impacts cannot be inherited beyond one generation. 'Epigenetic inheritance' has now been demonstrated in mice.[22] This could explain why Dutch women who were starved during their pregnancy in World War II had stunted *grandchildren*. In Brazil it is noted that brain size has been reducing in some poor regions over the past thirty years, because of dwarfism caused by malnutrition.[23]

Even simple causes such as iron and zinc deficiency resulting from the Green Revolution might have an effect (see Chapter 6). The impact is already apparent across whole populations – millions are affected – and many of these people remain in reproductive proximity. This cause could be compounded by many other adverse chemical factors, and then a degenerative psycho-social spiral, which could perhaps lead eventually to genetic regression in the brain.

It seems reasonable to conclude that, as our current brain is the result of millions of years of progressive evolution, any regression would also take millions of years. This may be so, or not. If rats are placed in an unstimulating environment the result is not just a vague behaviour change but a *visible* biochemical decline in brain functioning, within months.[24] This happens without any additional chemical threats or intergenerational impacts. Rats placed in stimulating or unstimulating environments become different from one another, and from their parent species, and the difference remains after just three generations.

The standard evolution theories maintain that it takes hundreds of thousands of years for significant genetic changes to become established in humans ('phyletic gradualism'), but now there are alternative models that suggest fast punctuational effects. John Eccles concludes, 'Major chromosomal changes may give the genetic changes requisite for speciation [the formation of new biological species] in a few generations of a peripheral isolate. Thus speciation may be dependent on gene regulation and rearrangement rather than on the classical point mutations that produce new genes in phyletic gradualism.'[25] Brain evolution may be less a case of make-or-break genetic change, and more one of a host of minute alterations which together then form an ineluctable driver of major change.

One argument against the possibility of regressive brain evolution is that progressive development only happened because of geographically isolated communities (peripheral isolates) within which genetic changes were preserved and perpetuated, and that communities of this type no longer exist. If this mechanism is not available for progressive evolution, therefore arguably it is not available for regressive evolution either. But do peripheral isolates need to be *geographically* isolated? Might *social* isolation have the same effect, particularly if a biological regression could be precipitated within a few generations?

People of low intelligence generally form a distinct cadre in contemporary society, even though geographically dissipated. In reproductive terms, they are usually, in effect, peripheral isolates. Because intelligence is a major determinate in the selection of a life partner, social pressures dictate that they will tend to intermarry, so genetic transfer could be 'isolated'. (But the offspring of people with 'clinical' intellectual disabilities do not necessarily inherit the disability.) In communities suffering EMID, especially if rural, the more intelligent members will probably migrate and those of lower intelligence will tend to be less mobile, which intensifies the isolation of the cadre.

Paradoxically, it is also arguable that social peripheral isolates are *more* probable in the large diverse human populations of the modern world. In small isolated communities, choice of life partner was dictated by the limited supply of available individuals within an age set. In this setting people cannot be so choosy on the basis of intelligence, so there will be a greater mixing-in of those with low intelligence. Put crudely, a man of eighteen is more likely to choose a pretty teenage woman with a mild intellectual disability than a forty-year-old who is a bit brighter, and this would probably meet with community approval on the basis of effective procreation. In a large, dense community there is greater general choice within an age set and therefore more probability that those of low intelligence will be left with no option but to intermarry.

These are, of course, dangerous waters, because the line of argument reflects that of the eugenics movement. But it was the eugenicists' *conclusions* that were wrong: much of their underlying reasoning was based on logical evolutionary understanding. The conclusions about EMID are about preventing a type of environmentally mediated injury, not a type of human being. Stalin advocated the feeding of the poor, and we would not deny the worth of the idea just because it happened to be a Stalinist belief. Logical lines of thought should not be discounted just because of the eugenicist taint.

If we accept an element of doubt – that current forms of EMID just might lead to regressive brain evolution in specific populations – the question is not whether we can reverse intellectual decline. That is just the dependent variable and an outcome for which there is essentially no cure. The problem is, could we reverse the environmental dynamics that cause this decline? Could we undo the Green Revolution, clear up the persistent hormone-disrupting chemicals and environmental lead, restore vital micro-nutrients to the soil or reverse a major driver of these dynamics, population growth?

Whatever the probability of regressive brain evolution, one message should be clear. Our brain now knows of its fragility within the ecosystem from the empirical evidence of contemporary medical science and ecology, and from the perspective of evolutionary theory. Why has millions of years of brain evolution given us the intelligence to know, but not the intelligence to act?

## Notes

1. J. Ashby and M. Kettle, 'Methods for assessing the effects of mixtures of chemicals', in V.B. Vouk and P.J. Sheenhan (eds), *Methods for Assessing the Effects of Chemicals on Reproductive Functions* (John Wiley & Sons: New York, 1987).

2. Tao Zufan and Wei Luxin, 'An epidemiological investigation of mutational diseases in the high background radiation area of Yangjiang, China', *Journal of Radiation Research* (1986), **27**, 141–50.

3. N. Kochupillai et al., 'Down's syndrome and related abnormalities in an area of high background radiation in coastal Kerala', *Nature* (1976), **262**, 60–1.

4. Chris Busby, *Wings of Death: Nuclear Pollution and Human Health* (Builth Wells, Powys: Audit Books, 1995).

5. Basil S. Hetzel, *The Story of Iodine Deficiency: An International Challenge to Nutrition* (Oxford: Oxford University Press, 1989), pp. 13, 175.

6. Mira Shiva, 'Environmental degradation and subversion of health', in V. Siva (ed.), *Minding Our Lives* (Kali for Women: Delhi, 1993), p. 62.

7. Hetzel, *op. cit.* (n. 5), p. 92.

8. Theo Colborn et al., *Our Stolen Future* (Little, Brown & Co.: London, 1996).

9. EPA, 'Identification and listing of hazardous waste, discarded commercial products, off-specification species, container residues, and spill residues thereof', *Federal Register* (1980), **45**.

10. A.J. McMichael, *Planetary Overload: Global Environmental Change and the Health of the Human Species* (Cambridge University Press: Cambridge, 1993), p. 101.

11. M.M. Velga, J.A. Meech and N. Onate, 'Mercury pollution from deforestation', *Nature* (1994), **368**, 816–17.

12. McMichael, *op. cit.* (n. 10), pp. 156–7.

13. James Lovelock, *Gaia: A New Look at Life on Earth* (Oxford University Press: Oxford, 1979), pp. 117–18.

14. Hetzel, *op. cit.* (n. 5), p. 4.

15. John Elkington, *The Poisoned Womb* (Penguin: Harmondsworth, 1985), p. 42.

16. McMichael, *op. cit.* (n. 10), p. 148.

17. William M. Stigliani et al. 'Heavy metal pollution in the Rhine Basin', *Environmental Science and Technology* (1993), **27**(5), 786–93.

18. Thomas Wynn, 'Archaeological evidence for modern intelligence', in R.A. Foley (ed.), *The Origins of Human Behaviour* (Unwin Hyman: London, 1991), pp. 52–66.

19. Christopher Wills, *The Runaway Brain: The Evolution of Human Uniqueness* (Harper Collins: London, 1993), pp. 8–10.

20. John C. Eccles, *Evolution of the Brain: Creation of the Self* (Routledge: London, 1989), p. 224.

21. Leslie Aiello and Peter Wheeler, 'The expensive-tissue hypothesis', *Current Anthropology* (1995), **36**(2), 199-224.

22. Irmgard Roemer, Wolf Reik et al., 'Epigenetic inheritance in the mouse', *Current Biology* (1997), **7**, 277-80.

23. Louise Byrne, 'Crippling poverty stunts Brazilian growth', *Observer*, 26 January 1992, p. 12.

24. Wills, *op. cit.* (n. 19), pp. 1–3.

25. Eccles, *op. cit.* (n. 20), p. 7.

# CHAPTER 10

# The Intellect in the Ecosystem

The potential hazards are ecological but the significant hazards are human. What, therefore, of the *outward bound* influences from Terminus Brain? What is unique about human intelligence and the way in which it functions in the ecosystem, which causes the self-threat that our brain now faces?

The brain comes into being, chemically interacts with the ecosystem and eventually biodegrades just like any other organism. From one perspective, this is all we need to know. Francis Crick makes the argument lucidly:

> *'You', your joys and your sorrows, your memories and your ambitions, your sense of personal identity and freewill, are in fact no more than the behaviour of a vast assembly of nerve cells and their associated molecules. As Lewis Carroll's Alice might have phrased it: 'You're nothing but a pack of neurons.'*[1]

But we are faced with the fact that if a brain were *just* a brain, we would not be in our current environmental mess. Even if 'nothing but a pack of neurons', it is a uniquely tenacious pack of neurons that changes its surroundings far more radically than its rival packs of biomass. The practical questions posed by EMID require a way to understand more clearly what the brain *does* to its environment, as distinct from what the brain *is* as an organism in that environment.

One starting-point is that as the human intellect changes its environment in a way that animal intellects do not, understanding the animal–human difference might identify what is unique about human behaviour. For many years, philosophers and scientists have tried to draw a distinction between human intelligence and that of animals.[2] It is not so easy. Work by researchers such as Jane Goodall constantly pushes back the divide, finding that animals can make and use tools, plan and communicate.[3] At Georgia State University chimps have been taught to communicate by sign language; one has learned more words than a 2-year-old child and can understand spoken English. A parrot at Arizona University has been taught to understand and use words to identify seven colours and different materials such as paper, wood and cork.

The job here is not to re-invent the human–animal debate, but simply to ask an applied question based on the fact that it is the human not the animal brain that is under threat from itself: what *unique* characteristics of human intelligence might lead to the environmental hazards that cause EMID? That animals and humans differ in their ability to create poetry, for example, seems of little direct relevance.

## The uniqueness of the human intellect

In *The Runaway Brain*, Wills determines two key characteristics distinguishing human and animal intelligence: 'the sheer amount of juggling that our brains can do', and 'the degree to which we can voluntarily override this continual sorting and prioritizing of new information' and concentrate on specifics.[4] These differences are very valuable insights, but are more of scale than of form. We are looking for behaviour that is so distinct that it bears virtually no relation to the abilities of the non-human eco-actors. Three basic questions seem likely to lead towards a better understanding. What is it that humans do? How do we do it? Why do we do it?

The answers to the first two questions are not complicated. Creating energy is the what; information processing is the how. We learned to harness fire and we learned to write about it. This is not just a matter of doing a few tricks bigger and better than animals – animals cannot do these tricks at all. But a few seeming exceptions to this generalization make it necessary to provide some tighter definitions.

Plants, animals and humans all create energy – for example, from food or sunlight – so energy creation itself is not unique. But this form of energy creation happens within the organisms themselves – it is *bounded*. Our special trick is to create energy in ways that are beyond the bounds of our own organism. We can build a windmill or a hydro-electric plant and walk away, and these entities will continue to create energy without our further presence until they break. And even then it does not require intervention from the same human (i.e. organism) to make them function again. Arguably, there are other non-human sources of unbounded energy creation – the sun, lightning, volcanoes and, with really bad luck, a monkey banging two flints together near some dry grass. But these eco-entities cannot control or manage the energy they create. The human uniqueness seems therefore that we can *make and manage unbounded energy sources*.

Unbounded energy creation is not the whole explanation. Had we stopped at learning how to make fire, there would probably be few environmental hazards. The next question therefore is: how did we end up using this ability in such a totalitarian manner?

Animals can process information, but only within and between themselves at an immediate point in time – their information processing is again *bounded*. Dolphins may well have exceptional mental maps of the ocean and be able to impart some of this knowledge to other dolphins in the vicinity. But they cannot record what they know for other, unknown dolphins to use. Humans can process information created by individuals without any contact with those individuals, and they can do this intergenerationally. We can record, discuss and more recently use the electronic media to process and manage our information in a manner that is for all practical purposes unbounded by our own presence or space and time. New information can be created simply by processing existing information, without any reference to the experience that gave rise to the existing information.

Again there is an exception that pushes us towards a tighter description. Arguably, all living matter can engage in unbounded information processing through genetic transfer. It is arguable whether or not this constitutes 'making' information, but even if taken as such, there is no subsequent control over what happens. It is our ability to *make and manage unbounded information processing* that seems unique.

The links between these two unique human abilities and the environmental hazards of modernity are all too obvious – the car, electric power generation, guns, population expansion and perhaps most significantly chemical synthesis. But these two understandings still do not provide the *why*.

However well we come to understand ourselves in relation to energy and information, it seems unlikely that we can put the energy-info genie back into the bottle, even if that were desirable. It is a genie that provides the more acceptable aspects of positive human survival – anaesthetics, electric wheelchairs, spectacles. It is the genie that creates the environmental problems, but also provides the means to solve those problems. We need to understand the why, because that is the route to changing the what and the how in a way that can preserve the good aspects of human life. We must understand our intellect not just in relation to human abilities, but also in relation to human behaviour.

## Human behaviour and pertinacity

Any extra-terrestrial intelligence viewing the current human relationship with the environment could be forgiven for diagnosing in its terrestrial peer some form of collective mental dysfunction, seemingly heading us for species suicide. What is the dysfunction, the human trait that drives us to use energy and information in such a potentially self-destructive way? The usual answer is 'free will', which can lead to a circular debate about the nature of free will, and the existence or wisdom of an omnipotent influence. But born of free will or not, we can still identify independent behaviour that might influence the relationship between intelligence and the ecosystem. The starting-point is a simple game of chance.

Toss a coin many times and record each time how it falls – heads or tails. The result will be a seemingly random pattern. But over a long period, the ratio will work out near enough 50 per cent heads, 50 per cent tails. There is, after all, some form of pattern. If we did an analogous experiment using an animal to generate the coin tossing, the outcome would be the same. The effect could be replicated by using a machine, or a natural occurrence such as the wind.

We could go further and devise an experiment that apparently permits an (untutored) animal to exercise its independent behaviour by choosing to *place* a coin heads or tails. The 'coin' might be marked so that it is possible for the animal to see a difference, perhaps dots on one side and stripes on the other. Unless there is an inherent reason for favouring one result (as there might be if colours were used), the outcome is likely to be a seemingly random, but over time 50–50, distribution.

Ask a human being to *place* the coin, and the result might be the same, but it might not. The outcome could reflect some form of plan resulting in a seemingly regular pattern – heads, tails, heads, tails . . . But this pattern could change at any time. The outcome could also be the persistent placing of one side – heads, heads, heads. . . And human beings can go one stage further. They might place the coin *tails*, heads, heads, heads . . . This removes any element of predictability that we might have concluded possible in relation to the previous outcome. Once we know that the individual *can* place tails, however many times heads is placed, the next time could well be tails.

Even in this very simple experiment, human independent behaviour, combined with the scale of our intellectual ability, can be expressed in tenacious outcomes that are quite distinct from outcomes generated by non-human intellects. Like unbounded energy and information, 'coin placing' is unique to humans because our intelligent behaviour stems from reason, not just causation. The consequence in relation to behaviour within a ecosystem sounds like a paradox. Non-human behaviour creates an outcome that, although seemingly random, is broadly predictable. Human behaviour can create an outcome that is *not* random, but therefore *not* broadly predictable.

There is a little-used word that would describe this uniquely human behaviour: we can be *pertinacious*, very or extremely (per) tenacious. The *Oxford English Dictionary* elaborates:

Pertinacious – *persistent or stubborn in holding to one's own opinion or design . . . Chiefly as a bad quality.*

The difference between human and animal tenacity becomes more apparent when we take these elements as a whole. A mule might be 'stubborn', but the stubbornness is unlikely to be 'persistent' over weeks or years. Any persistence certainly will not be intergenerational, which humans can achieve because of information processing. Few would argue that the mule's stubbornness derives from an 'opinion', but even if it does, it is unlikely to form part of an overall 'design', and it seems improbable that it is the mule's 'own' design. Humans are capable of persistence *and* stubbornness *and* having their own opinions *and* design.

Existential human suffering arises, in the Buddhist view, when we cling to fixed forms and categories created by the mind instead of accepting the impermanent and transitory nature of all things . . . Trying to cling to our rigid categories instead of realising the fluidity of life, we are bound to experience frustration after frustration.[5] Fritjof Capra, *The Web of Life* (HarperCollins: London, 1996), p. 286.

Some forms of behaviour are not necessarily closely related to intelligence – kindness, for example. Pertinacity is at the other end of the spectrum, characterized by and closely correlated with intellectual abilities. Pertinacity is distinct from obsessive-compulsive behaviour, which, in the sense used by psychologists, persists *against* the design or opinion of the person concerned, and affects individuals in isolation. An example is the obsessive behaviour of an individual who wants to be thin but continues to eat chocolate excessively.

As is usual with definitions of behaviour, we add a moral dimension – the outcome of pertinacity is usually taken to be 'bad'. The trait might well be seen to underpin many of the world's ills: genocide, fundamentalism, apartheid, witchcraft killings, China's Cultural Revolution. The word cultural is often used to explained such ills. A neat phrase from Clyde Kluckhohn – culture is a '*design* for living' – unwittingly makes a link between the definitions of pertinacity and culture. And cultural design usually becomes internalized as our 'own design'. Perhaps more ominous is one obsolescent definition of pertinacious, in relation to disease – 'not yielding to treatment'.

How might pertinacity constitute an extreme and adverse dynamic within an ecosystem? It seems plausible that the ecosystem will have more difficulty interacting with those persistent, 'coin-placing', non-random but broadly unpredictable human generators than it does with the non-human ones.

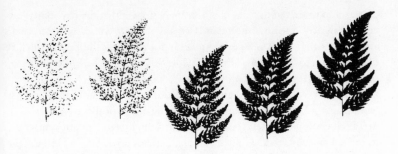

**Figure 10.1**  A result from Michael Barnsley's 'chaos game'.
*Source:* Michael Barnsley, *Fractals Everywhere* (Academic Press: Boston, 1988).

History tells us that we have been such persistent hunters that we hunt to extinction, such persistent gatherers that there is nothing left to gather, such persistent foresters that forests disappear, such persistent cultivators that the soil becomes uncultivatable. Stubborn and persistent behaviours such as excessive pesticide use, car addiction and unnecessary consumerism, while perhaps in line with a cultural design, all seem in conflict with ecological equilibrium.

An aspect of chaos theory suggests another intriguing possibility, and perhaps a deeper understanding. In *Fractals Everywhere*, Michael Barnsley explains a randomness technique, which he called 'the chaos game'. Among other things, the technique models natural shapes. In principle, the game just requires pen, paper and a coin to toss. James Gleick provides a lucid explanation.[6] You make up two rules, one for heads and one for tails. For example: tails, move two inches to the north-east; heads, move 25 per cent closer to the centre of the paper. Start anywhere on the paper, keep tossing the coin, and place dots at each landing point. If you ignore the first fifty results, the image – after you have made many, many dots -- will have a regular form. Replacing the pen, paper and coin with a computer makes the experiment workable. One of the most striking results from this form of encoding is in the shape of a fern leaf (Figure 10.1).

Many similar results led Barnsley to suggest that nature might be playing a similar chaos game, in the form of a biological encoding of information:

> *These images show complex blobs that are reminiscent of something small, biological, and organic. They make one think of the nuclei of cells; of collections of cells during the early stages of development of an embryo; of the process of cell division; and of protozoans.*[7]

Working along similar lines to Barnsley, John H. Hubbard made a comment which suggests that the form of biological encoding suggested by the chaos game is not restricted to plant life: 'I strongly suspect that the day somebody actually figures out how the brain is organized they will discover to their amazement that there is a coding scheme for building the brain which is of extraordinary precision.'[8] Perhaps God *did* play dice with the universe, or at least did not create it on the basis of 'dice-placing' behaviour.

A random 'coin-tossing' generator produces these results, not a human 'coin placer'. This seems to illustrate a striking distinction between the way in which ecological intelligence and human intelligence might impact on its overall environment, a distinction that perhaps provides a crucial insight into our conflictual relationship with the ecosystem. Ecological 'randomness' as a generator, plus the right set of encoded instructions, appears to create structure and order within which the ecosystem can maintain its equilibrium, because natural randomness is ultimately predictable in some way. Humans can act as a completely different form of generator, and it seems plausible that ecological coding schemes may not be able to cope with pertinacious human behaviour because it is both rigid and unpredictable.

If a human 'coin-placing' generator repeatedly placed heads, the result on Barnsley's computer would be a straight line. And even with the seeming randomness of the chaos game there appears to be one course of 'coin-tossing' action that would not work. If (using Gleick's rules, above) the first dot were placed exactly in the centre of the paper or on the line north-east of this, however many moves you make, the result is to go up and down that north-east furrow – there is no escape. The chance of a non-human 'coin-tossing' generator hitting on these starting-points is remote, but even in nature a few progeny are stillborn or defective. The human generator can work out the Achilles' heel of the system and, if desired, take advantage of it, deliberately carving out a straight line through 'coin-placing' behaviour. This image, a laser-like linearity, seems consistent with environmentally destructive human behaviour such as that which has cut holes in the ozone layer with CFCs. It also reflects the vision of the modernity super-vectors mentioned in Chapter 9 – the new fast lines from potential environmental hazards to Terminus Brain.

Not only does the encoding of the 'coin-tossing', non-human generator abhor straight lines, it also avoids exact replication. Fern leaves all have the same pattern, but you will never find two leaves of exactly the same shape. They perhaps become the random generator for the next round of the eco-chaos game. Conversely, humans are able to create designs for living that are static and repeated, and this linearity seems to be ecologically lethal. Persistent straight lines are rare in nature, but common in the human way of thinking. The broader relationships between our 'linear thinking' and environmental security are explained by Gwyn Prins in *Threats without Enemies*.[9]

Recall Christopher Wills's argument in Chapter 9, that the evolution of the brain may in part be due to a 'loop' – the environment that constructed the human intellect was the environment that the human intellect helped to construct. If this is correct, the pertinacity trait seems to represent an inherent flaw in the loop. This may have been so for millennia, but now the modernity dynamics provide the impetus for a large-scale effect. At the very least, the existence of EMID suggests that any notion that this loop will permit ever-continuing evolutionary improvement of the brain and its intellectual potential would seem now to be open to question.

The consequences of human tenacity, like other aspects of independent behaviour, are, of course, not necessarily adverse. There are grey areas. What, for example, is the difference between the violin virtuoso and the creator of leaded petrol – the Menuhin and the Midgley? Both might have arrived at their ends by something that could be termed pertinacity. The difference seems to be determined by two concepts, *dependence* and *cumulative* endeavours.

If we bring in the other two aspects of the uniqueness of human intelligence mentioned above – energy and information – one factor quickly distinguishes Menuhin and Midgley. The impact of Midgley's endeavour was highly *dependent* on energy and information processing to create and promote leaded petrol. Menuhin may *use* the products of energy and information, but he is not *dependent* on them. A modern violin may use metal strings and tuning devices, and even synthetic varnish, but violins can be made without these extras. While printed music (processed information) broadens the scope of musical endeavour, musicians can exist without a written tradition. One characteristic of adverse pertinacity, in relation to the environment, is therefore that it *depends* on energy use and information processing.

Music and motor cars are distinctive circumstances, so what about something less clear-cut? Pertinacious scientific endeavour may well have underpinned the development of both penicillin and the atom bomb, and both depend on energy and information. The former is unlikely to be seen as an adverse outcome; the latter makes the world less safe. While remaining isolated as laboratory experiments, both were essentially neutral in their impact on the world. It is the *cumulative* pertinacity of science, technology, commerce and politics that turned scientific understanding of the atom into the global threat as it now exists. Some new drugs may also fit this pattern – thalidomide, for example.

On the borderlines, the distinctions between positive and adverse tenacity are, of course, infinitely arguable. The difference is between tenacity and *per*tinacity. The per (the 'very') relates back to two earlier points. First, to those dynamics of modernity – very big, very fast and very mixed up –

which are both cause and effect of our contemporary behaviour. Second, to the two unique aspects of the human brain proposed by Christopher Wills: our intellectual capacity is very big and so too is our ability to focus within this capacity.

There is a third pertinent factor proposed by Chris Stringer and Robin McKie in *African Exodus*. Interestingly they argue, on the basis of a weakness rather than a strength of our intellect, that the brain's evolutionary pattern means that we are not able to comprehend and perceive very large numbers. One result is an inability to envisage the consequences of environmentally incongruous behaviour when magnified by large populations:

> We are the prisoners of a limited mentality, a handicap that prevents us from truly understanding numbers of humans greater than a few hundred. Our lack of large-scale empathy may soon kill us . . . As our technology becomes more sophisticated and speedy we face the prospect of simply being overwhelmed by it . . . As Eric Harth states in Dawn of a Millennium: 'Human beings are not wired for such speeds and informational deluge' . . . We had just enough brainpower to develop technology, but may simply have stopped short of the full evolutionary changes needed to control our creations.[10]

They continue with another conclusion by Eric Harth: 'Technology is *cumulative*, growing through the addition of many small contributions, while intelligence, the source of this steady growth, remains fixed.'[11] (Emphasis added.) How many people can truly envisage the consequences of the population doubling in forty years, or even of a doubling of car use in one country? This situation is compounded by scientific method. Richard Levins, Professor of Population Sciences at the Harvard School of Public Health, considers that the intellectual barriers to solving health and environmental problems stem from 'the reductionist strategy of Euro-North American science which chose the smallest possible object as the "problem", and then divided this into its smallest parts for analysis'.[12]

The human intellect will always create the Menuhins *and* the Midgleys, the tenacious and the pertinacious. Our hope for survival is that it also gives rise to human populations intelligent enough to judge between the two. And this seems to bring us full circle in the argument about the importance of protecting human intellectual resources against the threat of EMID. But that is from a *human* perspective — the perspective of the ecosystem may be different.

## From the ecosystem's perspective

We rarely ask: what is the benefit or otherwise of the human intellect to the ecosystem? When we do, the answers are inevitably human-centred. If a dolphin were writing about the place of human intelligence in the world, the story might have a different slant. There are four related questions which might help to develop an alternative perception.

Does the uniqueness of the human intellect create a form of behaviour and resultant modernity that is dysfunctional within the ecosystem, giving rise to EMID?

The evidence supporting this is outlined within this book. While individual studies may have weaknesses, taking the weight of evidence as a whole the idea seems hard now to dispute.

Could EMID reduce the *ability* of humans to perpetuate modernity?

Human populations with an intellectual ceiling of around IQ 70 would certainly not be able to plan and construct the dynamics of modernity, and they could not make and manage unbounded energy and information in the manner of their more intelligent peers. Even where feasible, their 'coin-placing' behaviour would almost certainly represent a random generator. There can be little argument about the *potential* impact of widespread clinical levels of EMID on modernity, only about the possible scale of effect given the limitations of current evidence.

Could EMID also act against human *behaviour* that perpetuates modernity, specifically pertinacity?

As, of course, relevant empirical work does not exist, we can do little more than contrast a few disparate concepts to explore this question. In Figure 10.2, the elements of pertinacity appear in column one, and in column two, terms describing sub-clinical EMID are placed against the elements *to which they are antithetical*. These terms come directly from Needleman's famous study of the effects of lead on children, so they *are* empirical,[13] and many studies from other sources would fit in a similar way. The juxtaposition suggests that specific forms of sub-clinical intellectual decline would act against the elements of pertinacity. Keep in mind that Needleman did not contrive his outcomes to counter a dictionary definition of pertinacious. Any link is either coincidental or indicative of a possible relationship between human behaviour and ecological behaviour that has not been considered.

Could the ecosystem defend its equilibrium by acting against modernity, through EMID?

However strong the indications, this possibility is difficult to accept, principally because it is taken to imply the existence of consciousness within the non-human ecosystem. Put another way, we would hate to think that

| 'Pertinacious'<br>(*Oxford English Dictionary*) | Outcomes of EMID<br>(Needleman) |
|---|---|
| **Persistent**<br>**or** | Not persistent<br>Day-dreamer<br>Low overall functioning |
| **stubborn**<br>**in** | Distractable<br>Hyperactive |
| **holding to** | Impulsive<br>Frustrated |
| **one's own** | Dependent |
| **opinion or**<br>**design** | Not organized<br>Unable to follow simple<br>directions/sequences |

**Figure 10.2**  Outcomes of EMID shown as antithetical to pertinacity.

the ecosystem is smarter than us. But it could be smarter than us without being so consciously. The unconscious ecosystem was smart enough to create our intellect, so why should it not be smart enough to control or destroy it?

James Lovelock provides a relevant insight into non-human intelligence:

> *Much of the routine operation of homoeostasis, whether it be in the cell, the animal, or for the entire biosphere, takes place automatically, and yet it must be recognized that some form of intelligence is required even within an automatic process, to interpret correctly information received about the environment. To supply the right answers to simple questions such as: 'Is it too hot?' or: 'Is there enough air to breathe?' requires intelligence . . . all cybernetic systems are intelligent to the extent that they must give the correct answer to at least one question.*[14]

Some bacteria move towards sugar; some move away from acid and heat; some can detect magnetic fields. There is new evidence that very simple forms of life can communicate and act cooperatively for common benefit.

Some bacteria live in communities and have a sense of their environment and of the existence of their peers. This quorum-sensing is evident in *Photobacterium ficheri*, a microbe that can emit light. The glow is very small or non-existent when populations are small, but when the population grows above a certain size, the microbes switch on and produce more light.

Richard Gregory, arguing a distinction between 'potential intelligence' (intelligence of stored knowledge) and 'kinetic intelligence' (intelligence of processing), provides another highly relevant line of argument:

> *surely, we should call natural selection intelligent. Indeed it is a very powerful kinetic intelligence that has discovered and invented answers and processes of life and mind that are largely beyond our understanding. Natural selection is the kinetic intelligence which over eons has produced the immense store of potential intelligence embodied in us. Babies do not have to invent muscles to move, or eyes and brains to see; these are already invented by the kinetic intelligence of evolution, and inherited as rich potential intelligence built up over countless generations.*[15]

Natural selection is an aspect of eco-intelligence, and one that is still operative.

It is therefore not implausible that other forms of intelligence can take us on and win. These non-human eco-actors, however simple, outnumber us infinitely and are, in evolutionary terms, playing on their home ground – that of maintaining eco-equilibrium through random but predictable 'coin-tossing' behaviour. If our brain is more or less 'nothing but a pack of neurons' and 'wholly chemically based', why should we be surprised that it is treated as such by the ecosystem that it is challenging?

But this scenario is founded on the view that there is competition between human intelligence and eco-intelligence. This may not be so – we might all be fighting on the same side. The 'survival of the fittest' need not imply competition at every level. It might simply mean a 'best fit' within a common environment, which is ultimately mutually advantageous. Eco-intelligence may well have created human intelligence 'in its own image', and both forms may be affected by environmental hazards in a similar way. But because human intelligence is more complex and more fragile, it will be affected first. Our intellect may represent the 'miner's canary' for an overall eco-intelligence of which we are a part. And as a fortunate coincidence, the demise of the canary would also entail the demise of the hazard.

Whatever the truth, it is as well to remember that human intelligence remains identifiable as the cause of the problem. If the human intellect is the enemy, or a traitor, or a lethal new recruit with a loose cannon, the need to deal with the problem is much the same from the perspective of eco-intelligence.

In his *Essay on the Principles of Population*, written in 1798, clergyman Thomas Malthus argued that the population would reach a size at which it would exceed the planet's ability to provide sufficient food. If writing now he probably would have added, 'and a size at which the planet will be unable to absorb the pollution that a large population creates', perhaps then conjecturing that the possible link between decreasing male fertility and pollution was another form of natural control. There is, he argued, an ecological glass ceiling on human population size. Currently the principle appears wrong because we have used our collective intelligence to increase the food supply and feed constantly growing numbers. But we also know that land degradation results from such intensive agriculture, and that this, together with the nutritional inadequacies of the food resulting from the Green Revolution, is causing intellectual decline. Perhaps the glass ceiling is a little lower, and less visible, than we think. The Malthusian prophecy may be taking shape and one of the first symptoms may be EMID.

But there is a more subtle scenario. Perhaps, because we can to some extent outwit the ecosystem when playing the simple Malthusian food resources game, eco-intelligence needs to operate differently – not just by curtailing the basic means of survival, but by curtailing our ability to play the survival game so well. The weakness of the Malthus vision is that it was entirely human-centred. His motivation for writing the *Essay* was to argue against providing support for the poor. He was not trying to save the planet. Denying food for the poor was apparently an acceptable line of thought for a Christian cleric in the eighteenth century, but permitting the ecosystem a point of view and the potential for intelligent behaviour was perhaps not.

Large populations do not *necessarily* threaten the ecosystem or themselves – the greater problem stems from how those populations behave. With half the current global population, and everyone behaving in the manner of the average New Yorker, human extinction would probably be near. *If* it could do so, it would therefore be logical for the glass ceiling to impede human ability and behaviour, not just population size.

If eco-intelligence solved the problem posed by modernity by curtailing human behaviour, it would perceive the impact of human intelligence as a collective force, not in terms of separate individual intellects. This would lead logically to an equation along the lines that the greater the population then the greater the sum of the collective intellect and resultant pertinacity, which therefore demands a crude reduction in the level of intellectual performance across the whole population. Just as the ecosystem has a ceiling on the amount of food that it will permit a collective population to extract, it might also have a ceiling on the sum total of ecologically extreme behaviour that it will permit us collectively to express.

There can be little argument that people who are seen as having intellectual disabilities usually lack the skills that have created modernity and its attendant threat to the ecosystem. Most significantly, they usually have restricted communication skills, and therefore their potential for information processing is limited. It would therefore be rational for eco-intelligence to *curtail* human intelligence. But there is a further possibility. Eco-intelligence may not just curtail our intellectual abilities and extreme behaviour to protect itself. Could it ultimately be far more subtle and *modify* the human intellect into something more compatible with the whole system?

It is interesting to look with an open mind at some of the characteristics of people we label as intellectually disabled. Some people *can* perceive the very large numbers that Stringer and McKie argue most humans cannot; for example, estimating accurately the number of ears of grain in a field of corn. This skill comes within the term *savant syndrome*, perhaps best known through Dustin Hoffman's portrayal in the film *Rain Man*. We often call people who display these skills autistic, but more accurately the syndrome is part of a continuum of human ability. Such people can also often see through complexity more readily. Research has shown that they can sometimes detect hidden visual patterns better than the general population – for example, to identify a simple geometrical shape, such as a pyramid, within a bigger, more complex, pattern. From some perspectives, 'intellectual disabilities' can start to look disconcertingly like the intellectual *abilities* needed by human beings if we are to behave more benignly within the ecosystem.

It is not just our disinclination to believe that ecological intelligence could be so smart that presents this line of thinking as science fiction. It is also that we cannot start to comprehend the magnitude of causal linkages that would need to be made for the ecosystem to exert this level of control over us. But is it that the number of linkages could not be made, or is it, as Stringer and McKie suggest, that we do not have a form of intelligence that can generate a perception of them? It is only the advent of the computer that has permitted us to perceive the countless links needed to construct those fern leaves in Barnsley's 'chaos game'. And the form of intelligence required for the basic encoding was very simple – like Lovelock's vision of eco-intelligence.

The conclusion from this line of thinking is not that eco-intelligence *is* currently curtailing or modifying our ability and behaviour to suit its own ends, but just that perhaps it *could*, and that this would be a rational means of defence against dysfunctional human behaviour. Our level of understanding may remain inadequate to reach firm conclusions about the long-term prognosis, but it is at least sufficient to recognize that there is an element of doubt about the potential of eco-intelligence. Exploring the meaning of that doubt could well be crucial to bringing about changes in pertinacious human behaviour which would prevent widespread EMID.

## Notes

1. Francis Crick, *The Astonishing Hypothesis: The Scientific Search for the Soul* (Touchstone Books: London, 1994), p. 3.

2. Harry J. Jerison, 'The evolution of biological intelligence', in R.J. Sternberg (ed.), *Handbook of Human Intelligence* (Cambridge University Press: Cambridge, 1982), pp. 723–91.

3. Jane Goodall, *The Chimpanzees of Gombe: Patterns of Behaviour* (Harvard University Press: Cambridge, MA, 1986).

4. Christopher Wills, *The Runaway Brain: The Evolution of Human Uniqueness* (London: HarperCollins, 1993), pp. 281–2.

5. Fritjof Capra, *The Web of Life* (HarperCollins: London, 1996) p. 286.

6. James Gleick, *Chaos: Making a New Science* (Cardinal: London, 1987), p. 236.

7. Michael Barnsley, *Fractals Everywhere* (Academic Press: Boston, 1988), p. 285.

8. Gleick, *op. cit.* (n. 6), p. 239.

9. Gwyn Prins (ed.). *Threats without Enemies: Facing Environmental Insecurity* (Earthscan Publications: London, 1993), p. 178.

10. Chris Stringer and Robin McKie, *African Exodus* (Jonathan Cape: London, 1996), pp. 227–8.

11. E. Harth, *Dawn of a Millennium* (Penguin: Harmondsworth, 1990).

12. Olga Wojtas, 'Call to reduce role of reductionist strategy in science', *Times Higher Educational Supplement*, 19 April 1996, p. 4.

13. H.L. Needleman, *et al.,* 'Deficits in psychologic and classroom performance of children with elevated dentine lead levels', *New England Journal of Medicine* (1979), **300**, 689–95.

14. James Lovelock, *Gaia: A New Look at Life on Earth* (Oxford University Press: Oxford, 1979), p. 146.

15. Richard Gregory, 'Seeing intelligence', in Jean Khalfa (ed.), *What Is Intelligence?* (Cambridge University Press: Cambridge, 1994), p. 15.

# PART V

# The Conceptual Environment

# CHAPTER 11

# Law and Regulation

Hit a child on the head with a hammer, causing an intellectual disability, and the act is seen as violent and there will usually be redress through legal channels. Drive a car using leaded petrol, causing intellectual disabilities in countless children, and the act is not seen as violent and the victims have no redress. Why do we not see environmental victimization as often prima facie criminal, violent[1] or representing a significant abuse of power by identifiable groups of people?

If our brain is to address the threat that it now poses to itself, it needs rapidly to rethink the taken-for-granted environmentally-mediated impacts on human well-being, and create new ethical understandings that can, if necessary, be operationalized as law. Part V should be the 'all change' at Terminus Brain: the turning-point at which we identify a new conceptual environment to organize our behaviour within the ecological and social environments in a manner that reduces the threat to the brain in its mobile bodily environment. The first step is to recognize *inconsistency* – in current conceptualization and consequent regulation – across geographical space, across time and between people. The eventual question is: do we need new special legislation, or instead should the ambit of existing personal injury law be developed?

## The law and EMID

How does the law protect the human brain? How do political convenience, power relationships and historical legacies influence the achievement of justice and the broader relationships between law and policy? Examples come from disparate sources spanning general brain damage, disability and environmental regulation. Legislation intended to redress or prevent environmentally-mediated injury falls into two broad categories: *case-related*, which is usually a political response to a disaster or particular threats; and *general*, which is more considered and aims to address a spectrum of known or possible hazards.

One of the more notorious examples of case-related legislation was the Bhopal Gas Leak Disaster (Processing of Claims) Act 1985. At the time this appeared to be in the interests of the victims, but the Act gave the Indian government the exclusive right to represent plaintiffs, compensation awards were therefore limited, and it prohibits claims from future generations. Implementation has been slow, ineffective and riddled with corruption. Compensation reaching victims ten years after the event generally amounts to about US$70 per person.

Do rich nations do any better? In response to high levels of disability after nuclear testing in Nevada, USA, there were two attempts at legislation, which displayed characteristics remarkably similar to the Bhopal Act. The first attempt,

> had it actually been passed by Congress, would have helped few if any [victims]. The radioepidemiological (probability of causation) tables upon which compensation would be decided were drawn up by the scientists formerly associated with the AEC and/or presently funded by the Department of Energy, National Institutes of Health, or National Cancer Institute, the foxes guarding the chicken coup. No independent (unbiased) studies were involved. This Compensation Act provided enormous loop-holes and escapes from liability, it freely applied concepts that understated the probability of causation.[2]

The later Radiation Exposure Compensation Act 1990 specifically excluded areas that have received high levels of fallout and excluded many cancers and other radiation-related illness, and there was 'no account taken of the legacy of cancers and birth defects in generations to come'.[3]

The UK Congenital Disability (Civil Liabilities) Act 1976 was a response to the legal difficulties experienced by people who were born with disabilities due to the drug thalidomide. It provides an interesting example of legislation intended to establish the rights of children injured *in utero*, and specifically includes radiation exposure. To its credit, the Act acknowledges time-latency, embracing 'predisposition (whether or not susceptible of immediate prognosis) to physical or mental defect in the future'. But despite its potential it has not been used much in relation to environmental victimization. Margaret Brazier concludes:

> The complexity of the Act has to be seen to be believed. Its failure to address the issue of causation, the greatest problem in any case of prenatal injury, has resulted in it being a largely useless and unused piece of legislation.[4]

Other forms of case-related legislation concern a specific cause rather than an event. Since 1938, a number of UK parents have argued that the vaccination of infants, particularly for whooping cough, has caused brain injury. Eventually the Vaccine Damage Payments Act 1979 was introduced to address these claims. While at last representing a clear acknowledgement by the government that a causal link exists, the effect of the legislation has been to limit the success of claims – four out of five fail. Access to medical records needed to prove a case can legally be withheld under the terms of the Act. The disability must be 'severe': 80 per cent, whatever that means. Even if claims under the Act are successful, payments do not exceed £30,000. The Act only applies to children officially residing in the UK, who were vaccinated in the UK. If a pharmaceutical company exported brain injury it faced no penalty at home.

The type of vaccine used in Britain and Ireland had been withdrawn in Germany and Sweden as unsafe. Research in Germany in the 1970s had found that the vaccine caused significant brain injury to one in 26,000 children, which was confirmed in a study of eight million children, and it was concluded that sub-clinical IQ deficit probably affected large numbers. Similar small-scale British studies had not detected this level of effect.[5] Why did the British government never accept the German evidence, when the research was done on a scale far greater than in Britain? The only scientific reason would be a claim that German and British children are genetically different, which is absurd. This glaring inconsistency in the acceptance of scientific evidence was probably not unrelated to cost and the lobbying power of British drugs companies.

In 1993, an Irish mother, a daughter of a bookmaker's clerk who left school aged 12, won a 20-year vaccine-damage battle with the Wellcome drugs company. She claimed that her son had suffered severe brain damage as a result of whooping cough vaccine made by the company. Having turned down the derisory £10,000 on offer through existing vaccine damage legislation, she finally achieved an award of £2.7 million for her son.[6] Victims can sometimes be better off if they ignore special legislation that purports to uphold their rights.

In this case, the vaccine manufacturer had not carried out a widely accepted 'mouse weight-gain test' on the vaccine batch that caused the injury. This was not required by law in Britain at the time, but the judge did not accept that the manufacturer therefore had no duty of care beyond statutory testing. He ruled that the test should have been carried out to the highest-known international standards. If this consistency precedent is eventually applied to environmental cases, the impact on public safety will be significant.

Workplace protection provides the main example of general legislation. Health and safety regulation in many countries is concerned with reproductive hazards, but it often does not stand up to close scrutiny. New regulations, such as those to check chemicals for potential neurotoxicity, are usually not retrospective. Therefore the older chemicals, which are often the most problematic, continue to be used untested. Discrimination on the basis of gender is often highly questionable. Maureen Paul discovered that the criteria used to restrict the employment of women of reproductive age in the USA 'bore little relationship to current scientific knowledge about the effects of particular substances or about the categories of workers truly at risk'. Neither lead nor radiation is formally regulated in a sex-specific manner, but often only women were prevented from working with these hazards, yet male-mediated effects are equally likely to injure a foetus.[7] As a result, women's employment prospects were restricted and the unborn child was underprotected from male-mediated reproductive hazards.

Workplace regulation often appears very questionable when viewed in relation to a whole population. The US Occupational Safety and Health Administration Lead Standard, for example, covers factories but does not apply to workers in construction industries or agriculture. US farmworkers have been excluded from the statutory 'right to know' in relation to pesticides, yet factory workers do have this right. Workplace protection under the Factories Act 1948 in India applies only to registered factories: most of India's labour force, significantly those in the informal sector, is therefore not protected. US industries involved in military contracts and operating on government land are exempted from oversight regulations that protect employees and the public by Presidential mandate. Some of these factories have been linked to significant increases in birth impairments.

Note how the US Occupational Safety and Health Act restricts its remit, when requiring exposure limits to ensure 'that no *employee* will suffer material impairment of health or functional capacity . . . for *the period of his working life* . . . [with the goal being] to provide safe or healthful *employment and places of employment*'[8] (emphasis added). Viewed another way, the Act implies: those who are not employees need not be protected; any health problems suffered the day after retirement are excluded, so don't worry too much about cumulative exposure; pollute as you like outside the place of employment. The child who suffers ill-health because of toxins brought into the home on a parent's work-clothes is not within the remit of occupational health and safety.

The high level of protection often afforded individuals inside a factory, as compared with that available to people living outside, is certainly not justified on the grounds of providing consistent protection to human beings. Legislation requiring fans to extract hazardous agents may protect the factory worker. Yet those who happen to live just outside the factory, perhaps by the extractor-fan outlet, might have no protection or means of redress. The motivation is not hard to imagine. Admitting responsibility for those inside the factory is limited and predictable. Admitting responsibility for those outside can open a floodgate. British health and safety law requires that employers 'ensure' that the general public are not exposed to risks to their health and safety.[9] But the potential to use this legislation to prevent or redress environmental poisonings is not fully exploited.

The artificial divide between the workplace and the external environment is a historical legacy, created by trade unions for the protection of exploited workers. The original aim of the unions was, of course, well intentioned, but the outcome now often represents the protection of one relatively powerful sector of the population at the expense of others much weaker. An environmental hazard inside the workplace could give rise to a dispute between, say, 2000 workers and 200 managers. If instead the hazard threatens 20 people outside the factory, those 20 may have to take on the combined might of the 2200 inside the factory, who will be supported by the curious alliance of trade unions and the government, all waving the 'protect jobs' banner.

It is very rare for damages to be awarded in relation to environmental pollution by a factory which affects people outside its boundary. The first UK case was in 1995. A woman who had been exposed to asbestos dust when playing many years earlier, as a child, near a factory now owned by the multinational Turner & Newall, was awarded £65,000 for resultant lung cancer.[10] The judge concluded that a 'duty of care' extended beyond the factory walls. At appeal, the defence lawyers realized that they could no longer argue on the basis of a distinction between a 'bounded' workplace environment and the 'unbounded' general environment. They then tried to construct a further boundary between what they termed 'guilty dust' just outside the factory wall, and 'not guilty dust' further away.[11] The absurdity simply demonstrates how any boundaries are meaningless if the genuine intent is to redress and prevent environmentally-mediated injury – and that those with vested interests will go to idiotic lengths to construct such boundaries.

It is not only in relation to workplace legislation that spatial restriction is questionable. The US Lead-based Paint Poisoning Prevention Act[12] aims to 'eliminate as far as practicable the hazards associated with unsafe levels of lead-based paint in housing'. Why only 'in housing' and not, for instance, in schools, where lead paint is common and children may spend more intense periods of time, or in hotels or hospitals?

Spatial inconsistencies are compounded by inconsistency in the way in which potential neurotoxins are tested. The US Congress report *Neurotoxicity* finds it of concern that, while the Food and Drugs Agency will test food additives by inferring low-dose effects on humans from high-dose effects on animals, pesticides are assessed in a way that 'accepts more general structured information in guiding neurotoxic testing'. And even in this sphere, while all pesticides are tested for general toxicity, not all are tested for neurotoxicity.[13] But even if the standards arise from erratic methods, we could at least ensure that the conclusions are applied equitably across populations. When researching *The Lead Scandal,* Des Wilson found that the (then) Greater London Council 'action level' for lead contamination was 5000 p.p.m. (parts per million) but its 'ideal safety level' was 500 p.p.m., and the Department of the Environment guideline was 2000 p.p.m.[14]

The piecemeal way in which law functions is indefensible if the intent is consistent human protection from environmental poisoning. Why does European law regulate heavy metals in air, water, land and plants – but not in food? The industrial use of mercury is usually controlled by statute – the use of mercury in cosmetics is not. Why can the UK Environment Agency control the incineration of toxic waste from the cement industry, which contains dioxins and heavy metals, but cannot prevent the same toxic waste being made into cattle feed? Why does government practice often not reflect the intent of government law? In Trinidad there is legislation to reduce the use of leaded petrol, but the state refinery does not produce unleaded petrol.

It is often even harder to recognize inconsistency at domestic levels because the construction of questionable boundaries often comes wrapped in regulations that appear helpful. In the UK, there have been state grants to householders for the replacement of lead water piping to dwellings. This seems benevolent, but the grant only covers the cost of replacement from the water main up to the house stopcock, not for replacing piping inside the house, which is probably the most significant hazard. All the water provider is doing is covering itself against damages claims that could arise in relation to the supply up to the stopcock. If the underlying intent were to protect the brains of British children, all piping would be replaced.

There is no reason why a nation cannot now have general environmental legislation that provides consistent protection for everyone irrespective of location, time or status. The South African Constitution of 1993, for example, states unambiguously: 'Every person shall have the right to an environment which is not detrimental to his or her health or well-being' (Article 29, Act 200, 1993). If the full intent of this Article is followed through in general legislation, it is hard to think why it should be necessary to treat the workplace, home, public buildings or anywhere else as a separate micro-environment. Perhaps those who drafted the Article did not intend cross-border responsibility, but 'every person' need not mean just South African citizens. The Article could well be taken as applying to the environment of those outside South Africa if it is affected by the acts of South African citizens.

If you drink American wine in America, the bottle will carry a warning that alcohol can damage the unborn child (see Figure 7.2). Drink the same wine outside the USA, and the bottle usually carries no warning. If US alcohol is a hazard to the unborn brain in the USA, why is it not considered a hazard elsewhere? If intellectual resources should be protected, surely they should be protected in an equitable manner. Any national policy operating to the contrary is, in effect, exporting disability.

Given that the vulnerability of the human brain is not known to vary according to nationality, inconsistencies between nations are indefensible. Des Wilson provided a survey of accepted levels of lead in paint (parts per million): USA 600; EEC 5000; UK 10,000.[15] It might be concluded from this that US brains are 16.6 times more vulnerable than those of UK citizens – or alternatively that British intelligence is 16.6 times less valuable to the British state than American intelligence is to the American state.

Why do we accept the pretence that each nation needs its own research to set standards? Scandinavian countries do not have stricter regulations in relation to solvent use because Scandinavian brains are more susceptible to the effects of solvents, but because research in those countries is very subtle and advanced in this area. So why, unless the science is shown to be flawed, should this not be accepted as a world benchmark? If there is need for evidence of the importance of international consistency, remember that Europe permitted the use of the drug thalidomide, while at the same time the US Food and Drug Agency did not. Eight thousand Europeans would now be a lot happier had there been a global precautionary principle.

Most significant at an international level is the blatant export of occupational hazards. The US Occupational Safety and Health Administration talks of 'conclusive evidence' proving that intellectual decline results from exposure to lead. So why does the USA not consider the evidence conclusive in relation to Mexican children whose brains are injured by US companies that operate, or benefit from, the *maquiladoras* factories? International inconsistency is often found in less evident guises. Pesticides banned in the UK and USA are used in Colombia, where they injure children working in the flower industry, yet the flowers grown as a result of using these pesticides are sold in the UK and USA.

There *is* a legal precedent for the cross-border protection of children. A few countries now have legislation permitting the prosecution in their home country of their nationals who sexually abuse children in other countries. An Australian and a Swede have received prison sentences for this type of offence. So why, if the consistent protection of children is the guiding principle, is it not possible to make similar statutory provision to charge industrialists who abuse children in other countries through poisoning them with environmental pollutants?

But the responsibility is not just in the hands of the perpetrator nations. Few governments of exploited nations take adequate measures to protect their citizens from external threats, because of the likely short-term financial loss. When will the exploited nations wake up and realize that importing intellectual decline is a very costly form of international trade?

Whether by intent or not, the South African Constitution – the section relating to the right to an environment which is not detrimental to health or well-being – could apply as much to the *absence* of necessary environmental agents as to the *presence* of undesirable ones. This reminds us of the other relevant area of general law, which concerns *absence*-EMID, specifically iodine deficiency. Once the basic right to life, health and well-being is established, from this logically follows instrumental legislation to provide the means to achieve these basic rights: for example, concerning water, food, micro-nutrients and health care. Many countries affected by iodine depletion are now passing legislation for universal salt iodization to redress the environmental deficiency: India, the Philippines and Pakistan are recent examples.[16]

But making a law does not guarantee that a problem is solved. Sometimes salt labelled as containing iodine, which is more expensive, does not. The manufacturers play on the fact that it is impossible to tell the difference without laboratory tests. A few years ago in China, salt sales were strictly controlled by the government. New open-door policies mean that unregulated producers now flood the market with uniodized salt which is popular because it is cheaper. The government official who is responsible for the iodization programme, Pang Peiyan, had to launch a campaign in 1995 to crack down on profiteers selling fake iodized salt. Open doors admit ill winds.

In general, responding to *absence*-EMID presents a problem of implementing rather than making laws. (And consequently, absence is a minor aspect of this chapter.) But one striking lesson comes from comparing the broad structural differences between law related to *presence*-EMID and *absence*-EMID – differences that at first sight seems too obvious to mention. Concerning *absence*, spatial consistency is not a problem – laws relate to the whole environment, not just to those in the workplace, school or home. Human consistency is not a problem – the law provides for iodine supplements distributed equitably across a whole population. Temporal consistency is not a problem – people of all ages benefit, including unborn children.

Why is there a difference? First, the provision of nutritional supplements carries none of the economic and political ramifications associated with preventing environmental toxins. Second, current iodine laws are not framed in the context of national historical legacies that create irrelevant boundaries. Third, in poorer countries laws redressing iodine deficiency are often supported by external aid, whereas anti-pollution laws usually are not. But there is perhaps another more subtle aspect. For centuries, our response to social problems has been epitomized by paternalistic charity: do something, give something. Redressing *absence*-EMID fits this ethos. But redressing *presence*-EMID requires us to *stop* doing things, and to *stop* 'giving' hazardous substances to human populations.

The latter is a new circumstance and consequently one that social theorists have not yet adequately addressed. For over a century, Marx and his followers have provided copious explanations about how the powerful deprive the powerless of vital environmental resources. The solution is, in theory at least, simple: do something; give resources equitably to those who need them. But in comparison there is virtually no social theory explaining how the powerful give to the powerless the hazardous 'resources' that they do not want. Even at a theoretical level the solution is elusive: stop doing something: don't give people resources that are the environmental equivalent of negative equity.

Our inability to equate doing and not doing goes beyond social theory. In 1948, Paul Müller gained a Nobel Prize for doing something: synthesizing DDT. Francis Kelsey of the US Food and Drugs Agency was the man responsible for delaying the licensing of thalidomide, and therefore saving America's population from its catastrophic consequences. He did not get the Nobel Prize for not doing something.

The difference between case-related and general legislation is unsurprising. Case-related law, drafted in the context of lobbying by powerful groups representing actual or potential perpetrators, contains countless caveats which limit liability and compensation, often to a point at which victims would fare better without special legislation. General law evolves without these direct pressures and so can take a more consistent view of human protection. But it is constrained by historical legacies leading to conceptual boundaries, which are meaningless in the light of modern environmental threats, but which also happen to coincide with the interests of those who might wish to restrict the efficacy of law.

If the protection of intellectual resources is accepted as a necessary goal, our increasing awareness of the problematic nature of EMID demands a reappraisal of environmental law to achieve consistency. But this is a problem that could provide the means to a broader solution. If we view the brain not as a problematic peripheral but as the logical hub of environmental law, EMID provides a conceptual focus around which many other aspects of human-oriented environmental protection would then fall into place.

## The cash-value of the brain

A glance at compensation awards resulting from medical negligence provides an important insight: the courts see the cost-consequence of brain injury as extremely high. In the UK, between 1992 and 1994, individual awards ranged between £1.5 and £10 million for brain injury at birth. Even convicted prisoners are treated equitably. In 1995, the UK Home Office paid £500,000 compensation to a prisoner given an accidental overdose of methadone as a treatment for drug addiction, which caused brain impairment. The point is not that a prisoner should not be compensated, but that the case presents such a stark contrast with our inability to acknowledge the deliberate acts of environmental victimization which lead to similarly debilitating forms of intellectual decline.

Brain injury is not acknowledged by the courts only in relation to medical neglect. Under the UK Congenital Disabilities Act, a child born with cerebral palsy and severe brain damage was awarded £700,000 damages against his mother, who drove recklessly and had a motor accident while pregnant.[17] A similar case arose in Sydney, Australia, where damages amounted to £1.3 million. It was, of course, the insurance companies who footed the bill, not the mothers, who were doubtless delighted to lose the cases. Even for adults there is a recognition of the cost-consequence of intellectual injury, although awards become age-related. In 1994, a British man of 48 who suffered brain injury from a traffic accident, leaving him totally dependent on his wife and able to communicate only by blinking, was awarded £900,000 damages, which was paid by the insurers of the offending driver. A 12-year-old who suffered severe brain damage after being hit by a speeding motorcyclist was awarded £1 million damages in 1991.

There are no prizes for working out why in some circumstances the brain is seen as so valuable yet in others that same form of injury is considered to be of no consequence. The brain is valued highly when the injury stems from an organization that can be made to pay up, and when cases can be restricted to a one-off circumstance. We currently accept that the brain is of little or no consequence when the injury might stem from the act of a powerful organization or when the likelihood is that large numbers may be affected and so the financial ramifications would be massive. The irony is that it is the high value we place on the brain in the first circumstance that gives rise to the low value we place on it in the second.

## The justice system and EMID

Court cases in relation to EMID are usually civil claims for damages, and most go unreported, so a comprehensive assessment is difficult. But the interesting point is that cases are being brought at all. The most notable was a claim against GPU Nuclear following the radiation release at Three Mile Island in 1979. A boy born with Down's syndrome nine months after the disaster was eventually awarded $1 million.[18] In 1990, a chemical plant in Pampa, Texas, was sued in relation to children born with Down's syndrome following an explosion and high levels of general pollution. This was the first case testing new theories that environmental toxins can cause Down's syndrome.[19] Three years later a group of parents working at the infamous Mexican *maquiladoras* took out a case against food giant Kraft and the battery company Duracell, because they believed that the link between children with severe intellectual disabilities and the factories in which the mothers worked was obvious. Gulf War veterans have started claims in the USA and UK not only for memory loss suffered by themselves, but also for birth impairments suffered by their offspring. In 1994, it was reported that Vietnam veterans in Australia were set to sue the government in a 'first-ever' case claiming that birth defects were caused by Agent Orange.[20]

In isolation, such reports may not seem significant, but they mark a novel turn to personal injury litigation, made possible by new scientific techniques that can support arguments about causal connections and EMID. From the perspective of history, we will be able to identify a clear era within which justice systems started to defend the brain against environmentally mediated hazards.

One of the most significant cases concerns the Chisso/Showa Denko mercury poisoning at Minamata Bay, Japan. This demonstrates a common injustice in such litigation: the delaying tactics employed by the responsible parties. In 1969, the Japanese government enacted a law for special compensation – 13 years after the first report of poisoning. Not until 1971 was the liability of Showa Denko to pay compensation finalized; the first court decision was in 1973. The eventual Pollution-related Health Damage Compensation Law was only enacted in 1974. Eventually, in 1987, the Kumamoto suit concluded with a finding that the national government should pay compensation for damages for the occurrence of the poisoning and for allowing it to spread. Finally, in 1995, 8000 victims were awarded £16,000 each, but on condition that they withdrew their cases against Chisso and against the government for allowing the poisoning. Chisso had spent 22 years fighting a ruling ordering it to pay £110,000 per year.[21] By the time they received their payment the victims were in their seventies: that is, the few that had survived.

Cases are starting to be brought in relation to less severe sub-clinical outcomes. Following contamination of the water supply with aluminium sulphate, in Camelford, UK, in 1994, victims complained of health effects including memory loss and feared the precipitation of Alzheimer's disease. The responsible company offered an immediate compensation payment, but only for short-term injuries, which would have precluded later claims concerning Alzheimer's. Eventually an out-of-court settlement of between £680 and £10,000 per person was made. The sums were small, but the acknowledgement of probable causation is significant.

In the same year a UK Industrial Injuries Tribunal made the first award to a farmer who had suffered loss of memory and motor control following exposure to organophosphorus sheep dip. The UK government had constantly refused to acknowledge any causal link, which is not surprising – for 16 years the use of the dip was a statutory requirement. Any sudden withdrawal of the chemical would have been a tacit admittance of liability. Because these chemicals are similar to nerve gas created for military purposes, their *prima facie* neurotoxic potential is not in dispute. For ethical reasons, they could not therefore be tested on humans in the course of medical research. But it *was* seemingly taken to be ethical to test these chemicals on a nation's farmers through legislation compelling their use.

Scientists who have worked on Ministry of Defence contracts point out that good data about the effects of chemicals related to nerve gas would have been available within government circles since the Second World War, but classified. The reason for classifying such information is national security. Environmental chemicals are now as much a threat to human safety as military conflict, so why are such data not used by governments to fulfil their original purpose – ensuring the security of their citizens?

Compare the cases affecting large numbers with that of the English cider drinker who claimed to have suffered permanent memory loss as a result of drinking from a mug with a leaded glaze in a pub. Lead exposure was ten times above the safe level, and the damages award was £55,000.[22] Why then do the courts not protect those within the 45 per cent of UK households where water arrives through lead pipes, exposing some to lead levels six times above the European limit? Why does the law not protect or achieve redress for the thousands of children who suffer because of leaded petrol? The responsible agents – the water companies and the manufacturers and users of leaded petrol – are readily identifiable.

Even if there is a high likelihood of litigation and compensation, this does not necessarily deter public poisoning. Penny Newman of Concerned Neighbors in Action documents one US instance:

> in a two-page handwritten note, a Gulf Resources and Chemical Corporation vice president in Idaho outlined estimates of how much Gulf would have to pay if it continued to expose children in the town of Kellogg to lead-contaminated smoke. The note's calculations were based on a 1970 lead-poisoning incident at an Asarco Inc. smelter in El Paso, Texas. The note begins, 'El Paso – 200 children – USD5 to USD10,000 per kid' and is

*followed by a reference to the Gulf operation indicating an estimated liability for poisoning 500 Kellogg children at 'USD6-7 million'. Even knowing the damage it was doing to the children of the area, Gulf increased the emissions from the smelter to cash in on the high lead prices of 1974. The children of Kellogg suffered the consequences. According to an EPA Inspector General's report, '. . . the blood-lead levels were the highest ever recorded. Of the 179 children living within one mile of the smelter, 99 per cent had blood-lead level over 40μg/dl. (The current standard is 10μg/dl.) The highest level recorded is 164μg/dl; 41 children had a blood-lead level over 80, the level established for lead poisoning.*[23]

The power of large companies is now such that it is all too easy just to cost the possibility of paying damages into the product price. Ultimately the only effective safeguard seems to be the use of the criminal law and the threat of prison against individual industrialists. People in Bhopal will commonly say that had a Union Carbide manager spent a few months in an Indian jail as a result of the mass poisoning, the safety standards of transnational companies operating in India would have changed overnight.

Although the UK has had a Control of Substances Hazardous to Health Act since 1988, it was not until 1996 that the first custodial sentence was handed out, for recklessly dismantling an asbestos building. South Africa provides another rare example of an attempt to use criminal law. In 1994, three managers at a British-owned company, Thor Chemicals, were charged with culpable homicide and 42 health and safety offences following mercury exposure within a factory. By 1992, one employee had died, one was comatose and another 'severely mentally disabled'. Twenty-six other workers suffered less serious effects.[24] The outcome was a derisory 13,500 rand fine and an acquittal on the homicide charges. But the interesting point is the almost unheard-of willingness of a government to use the criminal law against industrialists. This was probably related to the strong social justice ethos prevailing within the new post-apartheid government.

The main problem when using the criminal law is the need to identify responsible individuals. Managers who hold the relevant information will always close ranks to protect their peers, and corporate law aids them in this obfuscation. In theory it *is* possible to achieve a conviction against a company for corporate crime, if a 'controlling mind' of the company can be identified. But in the UK there has been only one successful case concerning corporate manslaughter, and that was not environmental.

There is a way around this problem. The precedent comes from Germany, in relation to law which regulates the export of materials or products likely to be used for military purposes by another country. Under the regulations, a *named* senior manager is held criminally responsible in the case of default. This principle could easily be applied to environmental liability. We tend now to forget that the original intent of laws giving companies a corporate identity was to enhance public, not private, interests. We need to challenge the more recent spin put on corporate law, which now pretends, especially regarding the environment, that original intent was the other way round. The norm in democratic nations was a point in history when public protection came first and those in the commercial sector were held responsible for their actions, as individuals, like any other citizen.

## Common law or special law?

In a very limited manner, the law *can* function effectively in response to EMID, but it is unlikely that current frameworks will ever permit it to do so adequately. The situation is hampered by the history of environmental legislation, which has evolved primarily to protect the environment, not us in it. It is hard to find any examples of an environmental criminal statute that *directly* protects humans – a law stating, for example, that if a toxic release injures a person then a case will be taken by the state in response to that offence. With the belated realization of the environmentally mediated threats to human beings, the approach has been to try to apply general pollution legislation, consumer protection or product liability law, or to stretch the remit of dated workplace legislation, none of which has been very successful.

The main message from this chapter is that special legislation seems to create more problems than it solves. Margaret Brazier concludes in relation to the UK Congenital Disabilities Act 1976 and the unborn victim: 'Ironically the common law duty owed to those born before 1976 has, too late, provided a more effective and comprehensive remedy than the statutory solution adopted in some haste.'[25] The alternative to special legislation, as Brazier hints, is the development of the centuries-old common law tradition in relation to personal injury. In general, there are two mechanisms resulting in brain injury: poisoning and assault. How might common law in these two areas address an environmentally mediated aspect? What are the conceptual blocks that prevent us giving the child who suffers intellectual decline from environmental toxins the same rights as the one who suffers in a very similar way through medical negligence?

In 1994, secret US papers were made public which revealed that, between the 1940s and the 1970s, mentally retarded teenagers at the Fernald state school, Massachusetts, were fed radioactive meals to permit military scientists to test the effects. Energy Secretary Hazel O'Leary argued strongly for compensation for these and numerous similar victims, including people who had been injected with radioactive substances.[26] A coalition of non-governmental organizations (NGOs), the Military Production Network, then broadened O'Leary's argument to include less direct military, environmental victimization on the basis that: 'There's no significant difference between someone who's been injected with plutonium and somebody whose [drinking] well contains radioactive elements.' This argument is difficult to counter on an ethical basis, but the US establishment could hide behind a problem of perception: the challenge to the view that poisoning must be an interpersonal act, that the poison must be administered and that the probable consequence is death.

Precedents for expanding prevailing perceptions come in relation to HIV/AIDS. In the UK, a woman infected with the HIV virus who injected her partner with her own infected blood faced trial in London charged with poisoning – 'causing a noxious thing to be administered so as to endanger life'. In this case the perception of poisoning was novel, because the 'noxious thing' was a virus, but not hard to accept because the act was interpersonal and life-threatening. Then, in 1994, in the French courts, the use of poisoning laws was considered when the national blood transfusion service deliberately delayed the introduction of a blood screening service for commercial reasons, with the result that HIV-infected blood was distributed. A charge of 'complicity in poisoning' was brought against ministers and others.[27] The usual perception of poisoning was therefore extended in three ways: the act was not interpersonal; it was an act of omission, not commission; there was only a potential, not direct, threat to life.

If poisoning laws can be invoked in these ways, why not in relation to toxins released from a factory waste pipe? The phrase 'so as to endanger life' could be taken to include the life of cells, or quality rather than length of life, or it might be argued that any form of injury or health problem endangers life to a certain extent. Useful legal precedents exist. Poisoning does not have to be deliberate, but can result from a reckless act, and the notion of 'administering' poison stretches to *causing* poison to be administered. UK poisoning law has been applied to spraying tear gas and to causing an escape of coal gas; both these example are very close to toxic environmental pollution.[28]

It might appear that all environmentally mediated poisoning would be covered by a development of poisoning law. But what about radiation? Although clinically it creates a toxic effect in the body, as an environmental agent radiation is not strictly a poison. What, too, about the lead in the domestic water supply of the person who declines to drink it and therefore does not suffer poisoning, just the threat of poisoning? How would poisoning law account for the environmental agents that are known to be toxic, but which can injure through such minute doses that their presence in individuals is near impossible to detect, or, in poorer communities, so costly to detect that cases could never be proven? Even if a toxin is identified within the body, how do we call to account an entity that contributes only a part of the overall environmental burden of that toxin – the lead smelter operating in an place that is already polluted with lead from petrol. In these situations we currently rely on laws that regulate the release of toxins into the environment, but which do not redress the harm they then do to individuals. It is in these areas that the criminal law concerning personal injury could become relevant.

Many years ago a Cambridge chemist decided to manufacture a chemical in the greenhouse in his garden, for sale to a local firm. Unfortunately, the process gave off a poisonous gas which killed his neighbour, and he was successfully prosecuted for manslaughter. Because the circumstances are local, the conviction does not seem very remarkable. But it provides an instance of the use of a standard criminal law in relation to an environ-mentally mediated toxin. At the time the case was probably not even seen as environmental; perhaps now it would be. If the circumstances had involved a chemical factory 50 miles away, the legal principles would be similar, but the scale changes our perception of the possible use of a basic law. If the law on manslaughter can be applicable to an environmental case, why not the next level down, the law on assault?

In 1992, a UK man who shook a neighbour's 22-month-old daughter 'so violently that she was brain damaged and crippled' was jailed for three years on a charge of assault causing grievous bodily harm.[29] It is therefore unproblematic to see brain injury as resulting from criminal assault, even when the brain was not directly the subject of the attack. So why can the principle of assault not be applied when the cause is environmentally mediated? It is now accepted that psychological trauma resulting from assault can constitute 'grievous bodily harm', so it should not be problematic to see intellectual decline, which can be assessed with greater objectivity, in the same way. The block is the perception that assault must be an interpersonal act involving direct physical contact, but is that the letter of the law?

Arguably, environmentally mediated injury embodies the common law elements of assault: force and violence. Technically, assault need not entail physical contact, and words alone may constitute an offence. An assault case has even been successful against a man who pulled faces to frighten elderly people, even though there was a glass window between him and his victims. The UK Crown Prosecution Service has now challenged the tradition that victim and victimizer should be in close proximity, by accepting that assault charges could be brought against a person who made hoax phone calls telling people that their relatives were ill in hospital. HIV/AIDS provides another incidence of innovative application. In 1995, a US soldier infected with the HIV virus was charged with assault after having unprotected sex with a female soldier who was unaware of his condition.[30] The offence was not sexual because intercourse was by consent. But the potential to infect with HIV involved force, not consent, and hence it was deemed an assault. It is not hard to argue that potential HIV infection could equate with a toxin in a water supply.

As it is written, even public order legislation might appear applicable to pollution. Under the UK Public Order Act 1986, there need not be an intent to cause injury – 'violent conduct' is itself an offence. Violence is an act that entails force, and force is something that cannot reasonably be resisted without a counter force. Many forms of pollution are less easy to avoid than a punch, so pollution arguably entails force.[31] Throwing a missile that could cause injury, but falls short, is specifically mentioned as being an act of violence and a public order offence. Spraying paint towards someone from an aerosol would therefore almost certainly constitute an offence, and a paint spray is not so dissimilar from the emissions from a factory chimney. The UK legislation does *not* require violence to be an interpersonal act. Behaviour that might cause a person of reasonably firm mind to *fear* violence is sufficient – the 'person' is hypothetical and does not need to be present. By analogy, the toxins from the factory chimney would not need to attack a specific individual for their presence to be construed as violent. Their presence as a force would be sufficient.

To provide another perspective, let us return to the area in which the law now finds it unproblematic to defend the brain: medical negligence. The way in which the brain, in its bodily environment, is injured by medical procedures mirrors the broader environmental paradigm. The hazards now accepted by courts are: the *absence* of necessary agents, principally oxygen, and the *presence* of harmful agents, such as the careless use of medical drugs. The latter is in effect poisoning, and one of the common forms of *presence* injury is careless use of forceps, which is technically an assault. The micro and the macro have remarkable similarities.

The point of this discussion is not to conclude that poisoning and assault law could simply be employed in cases of environmental victimization at the present moment, but to propose that it is more our historically bound perception of personal injury than the letter of the law that presents the idea as impossible. Put simply, the evolved perceptions would be:

- *Environmentally mediated poisoning:* the violation or attempted violation of the body by any human-generated toxin, irrespective of the adjacency of the source or likelihood of death.

- *Environmentally mediated assault:* a human-generated environmental *force* that has the potential to inflict harm on human beings because of its ineluctable nature.

If we could make a leap in our perception of personal injury, and evolve common law or make incremental legislative change, this would spare the need for a mass of new and potentially ineffective and inequitable environmental legislation in coming years.

## Notes

1. Christopher Williams, 'Environmental victimization and violence', *Aggression and Violent Behaviour* (1996), **1**(2), 191–204.

2. Re: part of the Senate Bill s. 1483.

3. Public Law 101–426; amended in Public Law 101-510, ss. 3139–3141.

4. Margaret Brazier *Street on Torts* (Butterworths: London, 1993), p. 196.

5. Neville Hodgkinson, 'Mother wins 20-year battle against drug giant', *Sunday Times*, 25 April 1993.

6. *Ibid*.

7. M. Paul, C. Daniels and R. Rosofsky, 'Corporate response to reproductive hazards in the workplace: results of the family, work, and health survey', *American Journal of Industrial Medicine* (1989), **16**, 267–80.

8. 29 USC.651 *et seq.*

9. Health and Safety at Work Act 1974, s. 3(1).

10. Jason Bennetto, 'Cancer sufferer awarded £65,000 in asbestos test case', *Independent*, 28 October 1995, p. 6.

11. 'Cancer from dust is like lottery', *Independent*, 27 March 1996, p. 8.

12. 42 USC.4801 *et seq.*

13. US Congress (OTA). *Neurotoxicity: Identifying and Controlling Poisons of the Nervous System* (Government Printing Office: Washington, DC, 1990), pp. 18–19.

14. Des Wilson, *The Lead Scandal* (Heinemann: London, 1983), p. 61.

15. *Ibid.*, pp. 61–2.

16. Rose Nathan, *Food Fortification Legislation and Regulation Handbook* (PAMM, Emory University: Atlanta, 1995).

17. O. Bowcott, 'Award for injury to unborn child', *Guardian*, 20 May 1992, p. 20.

18. Tim Cornwell, 'Roses in a nuclear garden', *Observer*, 12 September 1993, p. 12.

19. Keith Schneider, 'Birth defects and pollution: issue raised in Texas town', *New York Times*, 15 April 1990, p. 14.

20. Christine Wilson, 'Agent Orange and Vietnam veterans', *Pacific Research* (1994), November, 42–43.

21. Robert Guest, 'Tokyo final offer to poison victims', *Daily Telegraph*, 6 November 1995, p. 16.

22. Gary Younge, 'Lead in mug poisoned pub cider drinker, court is told', *Guardian*, 17 January 1996, p. 5; 18 January 1996, p. 7.

23. Penny Newman, 'Killing legally with toxic waste: women and the environment in the United States', in Vandana Shiva (ed.), *Minding Our Lives: Women from the South and North Reconnect Ecology and Health* (Kali for Women: Delhi, 1993), p. 49.

24. Richard Meeran, 'Legal accountability for the transfer of hazardous technology by corporations', unpublished paper, Leigh Day & Co Solicitors, London, 1994.

25. Brazier, *op. cit.* (n. 4), p. 196.

26. Jill Smolowe, 'The widening fallout', *Time*, 17 January 1994, pp. 30–1.

27. Julian Nundy, 'French courts summon blood scandal ministers', *Independent*, 22 September 1994, p. 11.

28. *Halsbury's Laws of England*, Vol. 11, part 1 (Butterworths: London, 1993), para. 475.

29. 'Baby crippled', *Guardian*, 12 May 1992, p. 2.

30. 'Aiding the virus', *Telegraph* (Calcutta), 15 December 1995, p. 3.

31. Williams, *op. cit.* (n. 1).

# CHAPTER 12

# The Science–Law Mismatch

When dealing with radiation, the UK Congenital Disabilities Act fails to make a distinction between effects on men and women *after* conception. It does not need a nuclear physicist to work out that dad could be passed through the core of a nuclear reactor after conception, without causing genetic harm to his progeny. At the end of centuries of wonderful science, it seems that we still have lawmakers who do not know that it is women who have babies.

In the laboratory, the scientist is judge and jury – the natural world provides the evidence. In court, science becomes the evidence – natural common sense becomes judge and jury. The aim of scientific method is to create a replicable process of investigation. The method of court investigation expressly precludes repeating the process unless it is shown to be flawed. Liona Salter terms the difference 'truth seeking' within science, and 'justice seeking' within the courts.[1] What are the relevant differences between the conceptualizations of science and law, and how might these impede an appropriate legal response to EMID?

The outcomes of the mismatches are apparent on two levels. First, they intrude on the technical execution of justice within a courtroom. Second, they display how inconsistent and illogical our standards are in relation to human protection in general. This is not evident because it seems incorrect to make formal comparisons between science and law, as they appear so dissimilar – you cannot compare apples and oranges. But comparisons can be made between anything, if an area of commonality upon which to base analysis is identified. Between law and (protective) science, the commonality is the shared purpose of public protection.

There is a long way to go before the fit between science and law is adequate to provide optimum protection for human beings in relation to environmentally mediated injury. But we can at least make a start by acknowledging some of the problems.

## Medicalized injustice

The child who is hit on the head is seen as a justice problem, with medicine doing what it can to cure the consequences. The child who suffers brain injury from lead poisoning is just a medical problem. Courts are not places to deal with medical problems, and so most environmentally mediated injury, particularly EMID, goes unredressed. Why this skewed perception?

Medical terminology is one reason. For many years medical textbooks have made a distinction between a 'birth defect' which is organic in origin, such as Down's syndrome, and a 'birth injury' which has a physical cause, such as the careless use of forceps at birth. An environmentally mediated impact does not fit this distinction. Radiation exposure may cause an organic 'defect' in medical terms, but in justice terms it should be seen as an injury.

To describe an injury as a defect could well have a subliminal effect on a jury, softening the perception of the event. But of equal importance, to label any victim as a 'defect' is demeaning and probably upsetting for family, which adds to the oppressive burden on those bringing cases to court. Courts would not get away with language of this nature if the description was of a woman who had been raped.

The more general use of medicalized discourse provides another level of obfuscation. Incidents such as the so-called Japanese 'oil disease' (*yusho*) and 'Minamata disease' are not diseases in the usual sense of the word. They can be neither caught nor cured, and are more correctly public poisonings. One academic paper mentioning *yusho* states that a 'similar *outbreak* had occurred in Japan in 1968'.[2] What is meant by an 'outbreak' of poisoning? The image this creates is of a causal dynamic within a community, yet the opposite is the truth.

The introduction to a glossy publication from the Japanese government, *Our Intensive Efforts to Overcome the Tragic History of Minamata Disease*, wraps an environmental crime in a shroud of medicalized analogy:

> Minamata **Disease**, which is a tragic experience of pollution caused **health damage** in Japan, was first discovered in 1956 . . . In 1965, another similar epidemic occurred . . . Since the first **outbreak** of the disease, research effort to investigate the causal agent has been made . . . As of 1991, have been certified almost three thousand Minamata **Disease patients** . . . Due to the **therapeutic** and protective measures taken after the discovery of the **disease**, Minamata **Disease** no longer seems to occur in Japan.[3] (emphasis added)

How do 'therapeutic . . . measures' relate to preventing the spread of mercury poisoning, the effects of which are not infectious and cannot be transmitted to others? Treating the victim of a snake bite does not protect other people – to achieve that you need to deal with the snake.

Medicalized language is perpetuated uncritically throughout the world. This is a very convenient outcome from the perspective of the perpetrator, and probably not altogether by chance – sanitized terminology may well influence a court. The perception if a lawyer talks of 'a defective baby with Minamata disease' becomes very different if the same circumstance is described as 'a baby who suffers brain injury due to poisoning by a toxin released from the Chisso factory.' It is not just that a court may be influenced, but that medicalized discourse deters us from even thinking of taking cases to court.

## Proof and uncertainty

The conventional notion of proof within experimental science is that it is only possible to establish a *negative* relationship. Popperian deductive method maintains that however many times a positive relationship holds, there can be no certainty that it will hold the next time. Theories can therefore only be falsified, not verified. In contrast, a court will only ever prove a *positive* relationship between events: guilty. A 'not guilty' verdict does not mean that a court has proven a negative relationship: that the accused is innocent. It simply means that it could not establish guilt. So when the judge asks the scientist, 'Does X cause Y?', the scientist who says 'Yes' is technically saying, 'I cannot prove that it does not.' This negative proof might then be taken as evidence favouring a positive court finding: guilt. These are clearly two opposite conceptual approaches, yet there has been little attempt to reconcile the difference or consider its importance.

Even when science can express its conclusions in the form a court might recognize, the degree of certainty is very different. The scientist will be talking of a 95 per cent degree as opposed to the (notional) 51 per cent 'balance of probabilities' required in a civil case. Even this seemingly impeccable 95 per cent figure masks broader uncertainties revealed by comparing a range of scientific certainties. Conclusions from separate sources concerning carbon dioxide emissions and global warming show a 50 per cent variation, for example.

The *Nordic Criteria for Reproductive Toxicity*[4] provide a typical example of the phraseology associated with scientific certainty.

*The substance:*

1   *is considered to pose a reproductive hazard to humans.*

1A   *is toxic to human reproduction.*

1B   *should be regarded as toxic to human reproduction.*

2   *is possibly toxic to human reproduction.*

3   *is not classifiable as to its reproductive toxicity to humans.*

How does this help when a judge asks simply, 'Could this substance have caused this child's birth impairments or not?' Even group 3, which sounds clear-cut, conflates substances for which there is evidence of their safety and those for which there are no data.

Scientific proof tends to deal with single causal relationships, but courts, particularly in environmental cases, must cope with multiple cause and effect. The words of the judge who accepted that causation would be sufficiently proved if it was shown that the negligent act was 'at least a material contributory cause' of an injury is not speaking the same language as the biologist who understands how a particular chemical causes a particular effect in a particular type of mouse under a particular set of circumstances.

Another similar judgement concluded, 'although the doctors cannot identify the process of causation scientifically there seems to be nothing irrational in drawing inference, as a matter of common sense'.[5] This is how a court might determine responsibility for a brain injury, yet drawing an inference from common sense is probably not how a brain surgeon would decide that a risky operation was necessary to mitigate that injury. And that same brain surgeon may be the expert witness in court.

The core of this mismatch stems from the question: who makes the decision that matters? At the present time scientists and justice systems both believe that it is the responsibility of the other to say conclusively what is dangerous and what is not.

## Consistent caution

The purpose of criminal justice is the protection of human beings; the protective sciences would make the same claim. But if we look at how the courts and science attempt to maintain this common purpose, when there is no proof and no certainty, the inconsistency is significant.

So far, regulators have generally accepted the 'innocent until proven guilty' maxim in relation to the testing of potentially hazardous chemicals. Perhaps this is because there is a sense that this reflects how courts operate. But there *is* a circumstance in which courts will treat suspects as if they are guilty.

Courts rarely make immediate judgements when faced with defendants who have been arrested and charged but who have not pleaded guilty. There is an interim period of uncertainty when guilt has not been tested or proven, and this poses the problem of what to do with an accused person during this time. It would seem wrong to let a possible murderer go free just after arrest, yet it appears contrary to natural justice to detain a person whose guilt has not been proven. Those not familiar with courts are often surprised at their powers in this circumstance. Following a simple set of criteria – for example, the likelihood of further offending, or the seriousness of the alleged offence – people who are technically innocent can be refused bail, and held on remand in prison, perhaps for many months, awaiting trial. The decision is made on the basis of a brief *prima facie* case, often outlined in a few minutes. No witnesses are heard and the defendant cannot directly challenge the assertions made by the prosecution. We accept that this precautionary principle is necessary for the sake of protecting the public, even though it might, and often does, lead to injustice against the suspect.

Now compare the treatment of 'suspect' chemicals. By complete contrast the public can be exposed to a new chemical, in relation to which there is *prima facie* evidence that it poses a hazard, simply because its guilt has not been tested. Pesticides (for example those related to military nerve gas) clearly pose a *prima facie* neurotoxic threat – that is exactly what they are designed to do. Yet they are often released into the public arena with little or no testing.

We can keep the human threat in prison before we have proof of guilt, but we can let the chemical threat loose on the public and test its guilt. Remanding the chemical would pose no possibility of a breach of civil liberties; refusing bail to the defendant may. Human injury may result from a wrong decision in either sphere, and probably on a far greater scale in relation to the chemical. No single criminal, working alone, could ever match the harm caused by the single chemical thalidomide: major injuries to 8000 people. And remember that in this instance the USA did keep the drug safely 'on remand' while Europe let it out 'on bail'. The argument is not for a life sentence, just that chemicals should be put 'on remand' until the case for releasing them has been fully assessed.

But even this style of argument is playing into the hands of the perpetrator. We are not really talking about suspect chemicals – we are talking about suspect industrialists, and 'remanding' the chemical poses a threat to the profits of powerful companies. If the response to the company that wished to expose the public to an untested chemical were logical – OK, but we will hold the board of directors on remand until the chemical is proven not guilty – the world would certainly be a lot safer.

Looking more broadly, even judges appear to accept a major conceptual inconsistency when there is a *prima facie* case that a particular environmental exposure may be harmful. A judge presiding over a public inquiry, hearing technical evidence from scientists, might rule that the low probability of one *theoretical* death or injury per million, as the result of potential exposure to an environmental toxin or radiation, is an 'acceptable' risk, and therefore the pollution (for example, low-level radiation) can be permitted. Yet if, at a future date, the same judge were hearing a case about an *actual* death or injury arising from the very same exposure, the low probability of that circumstance happening would never be accepted as a defence. The judge presiding over an inquiry may conclude that theoretical death or injury can be traded on a cost–benefit basis, but in a court hearing would always maintain that actual death or injury cannot.

## Protecting the vulnerable human

The scientist who claims in court that a certain level of toxic exposure poses no hazard because it is below a 'safe level' does so in relation to the scientific notional 'average human' – a concept that the court does not formally recognize. As explained in Chapter 4, those who may have specific vulnerabilities – because of, for example age, gender or clinical status – are at greater risk than this notional 'average human', and any assessment of the extent of that extra risk is usually only a guess.

If a court were considering the case of a victim of a minor assault, who died because a single punch triggered a vulnerability such as a heart condition, the assailant could still be convicted of unlawful killing. It would not be a defence for the attacker to claim that such a punch would not have killed an 'average human'. (It might mitigate the sentence.) In relation to general personal injury, the court affords equitable protection on the basis of the *most* vulnerable human, not a theoretical 'average human'.

By contrast, in relation to environmentally mediated poisoning, the 'average human' is currently an acceptable construct, even in court. If there were an adverse impact of a toxin on a 'below average human', this might *not* be construed as an offence because the exposure happened to be below a theoretical 'safe level'. In other words, the individual's vulnerability is seen as the cause of the injury, not the poisoning.

We can go a stage further. In the case of the minor assault the sentence might be increased if the vulnerability could have been recognized by the perpetrator: for example, if the victim were elderly. Those who introduce toxins into our environment often *do* know that they can have adverse effects on vulnerable people.

Now the full paradox emerges. In many cases of environmentally mediated injury, because science *does* know that some people are vulnerable, this knowledge is used in court to support the *defence* of the perpetrator. (The notion of an 'average human' acknowledges that there must be some below this average.) In all other spheres of human injury, knowledge of vulnerability is used to support the *prosecution* of the perpetrator.

## Population versus individual logic

The use of epidemiological studies in court is a contentious area in which science–law misunderstandings affect the technical execution of justice. The reason is that the difference between population logic (epidemiology) and individual causation is often neither admitted nor understood in courts; nor is it fully recognized that EMID poses unique problems.

Epidemiology might be used to help a court to determine if a particular cause were linked to a particular outcome – did radiation from this power station cause this case of Down's syndrome? Epidemiology is related to what is termed the 'normal condition' of a human being within the philosophy of causation in law,[6] although this is not acknowledged. For example, common sense tells us that a black eye is not a 'normal condition', and therefore if someone is punched in the eye, the change (the blackness) from the normal condition is caused, for the purposes of the court, by the punch. This approach works well with black eyes, and even cancer, but it breaks down fast when the change from a normal condition is intellectual decline caused by environmental agents.

Our 'normal condition' is without black eyes and cancer. But now it is not without body burdens of lead, PCBs and other human-made environmental neurotoxins, and in some settings probably not without some level of intellectual decline. Outside the courts epidemiology recognizes this fact, yet when epidemiology enters the courtroom we try to apply the simple black-eye logic to complex environmental causation and an indeterminate outcome.

In terms of an *individual*, disability is *not* usually seen by a court as a 'normal condition', and this is reflected in court discourse. For example, in one UK case, judges stated 'that the applicant was born with congenital characteristics *not present in a normal child*. These include profound mental handicap; deafness; microcephally; and various *abnormal* physical characteristics.'[7] (Emphasis added.) But in terms of any human *population*, disability *is* 'normal'. In any country, about 3 per cent of a population will be defined as having an intellectual disability. The difficulty for the court is to prove that the 'normal condition' of a particular disabled child would have been without disabilities had he or she not been exposed to a particular environmental agent. By using epidemiology we try to prove individual causation by using the logic of group causation – individual (court) logic holding that disability *is not* a 'normal condition' but group (scientific) logic holding that disability *is* a 'normal condition'.

The result is confusion between the way in which laws are framed, judgements are made and cases are argued. For example, the UK Congenital Disabilities Act 1976 specifically relates to environmental agents which 'affected either parent of the child in his or her ability to have a *normal* child'. Yet a case might be defended on the basis that the individual disability was normal because, based on group logic (epidemiology), a certain level of disability is normal.

From an epidemiological study, it might be possible to argue a *general* victim status if a community in the vicinity of a lead smelter had a 7 per cent incidence of intellectual disability, because the norm is 3 per cent. But it is not possible to identify exactly who, as individuals, constitute the 4 per cent victims. Other evidence is needed: for example, showing high blood lead levels. But this is not conclusive, because the understanding of what is 'high' derives from the questionable 'safe' levels and 'average human' construct, discussed above.

Victims with a pre-existing intellectual disability pose a further complication. They might also have high blood lead levels, but lead was not the cause of their initial disability. It would be wrong, however, automatically to deny them victim status, because the lead may well have worsened their condition. And this conundrum gets even more confused if we are talking about *in utero* injury, which may coincide with a naturally occurring impairment in the foetus.

One solution is to accept the extended notions of environmentally mediated poisoning and assault, discussed in Chapter 11: in other words, to determine the offence principally in relation to the nature of the act (or omission) of the perpetrator, rather than by its apparent effect on the victim.

Defence lawyers often argue their case by making comparisons with epidemiological studies elsewhere. They might claim that an individual birth within a cluster of five Down's syndrome births near a nuclear power station is 'naturally occurring', because clusters of five occur in other areas where there is no apparent exposure to radiation. It is rarely asked what caused the other clusters – are they truly a 'natural' condition? In fact, to prove that these clusters were natural would be impossible because scientific knowledge of the causes of Down's syndrome cannot currently provide the answer. 'Natural' usually just means that the cause of general clustering is not known.

Although improbable, it could even be proposed that all Down's syndrome clusters (not cases) have been caused by human-created radiation. Our records of Down's syndrome clusters go back only a few decades, and we have only recently established that background radiation from human sources such as weapons testing and releases from nuclear power stations does seem to cause such clusters. Since the 1950s everyone has been exposed to this source of radiation. Some groups have been more exposed than others, but there are now few completely uncontaminated control groups to permit definitive conclusions about natural clusters.

Let us take a more graphic example to illustrate this point. If we were comparing clusters of children with missing limbs, it might appear reasonable to argue, on the basis that clusters of six such children were common throughout a country, that a cluster of five in a particular location could not be attributed to a local environmental toxin. But we could add another piece of information that would present the argument in a completely different light: that we were talking about Cambodia, where the loss of limbs due to mines is very common. The Cambodia factor completely changes the argument, but only because the cause of the comparison–group clusters becomes so clear and comprehensible given the extra information.

In 1995, there was concern in the UK that unusual clusters of children born with missing limbs might have been caused by environmental toxins such as dioxin. Epidemiologists concluded that the clusters were 'most probably due to chance'. This is no surprise, but the revealing part of the conclusion was buried in a qualification: 'pending a fuller understanding of limb development in unborn children'.[8] Unlike landmines, the 'natural' cause of clusters among comparison groups may simply be beyond current comprehension.

Even if epidemiologists could show beyond doubt that clusters of, say, a particular cancer throughout a country were truly natural, this would not prove conclusively that a single incidence of that cancer near a factory was not caused by the factory. It diminishes the probability – but only from the perspective of population logic.

In a discussion of anophthalmia (children born with no eyes), which could have been caused by pesticides, Ruth Gilbert provided an illuminating argument, and her conclusions may surprise other epidemiologists:

> *Future research should be designed to benefit those at risk, and studies of clustering may not achieve this. Clustering could be consistent with fetal exposure to pesticides, pesti-virus, or other environmental agents; genetic susceptibility to specific environmental agents; or even a genetic cause if affected family members lived in the same area. Conversely,* the absence of clustering would not provide evidence against an association with a specific environmental factor, *particularly if exposure to that factor is widespread.*[9] *(emphasis added)*

At the time at which this was written, epidemiological evidence was being used by the pesticide manufacturers to refute a causal link, and no court had ever accepted a link between an airborne pesticide and birth impairments. Then, in 1996, a jury in Miami awarded US$4 million damages to a boy born with anophthalmia after his mother had been exposed to a fungicide during pregnancy. One of the key pieces of evidence was from new experimental research showing that even minute doses could produce serious damage.[10] Epidemiology tends to favour the case for the defence, not because it is methodologically flawed but because it is limited, misused and misunderstood.

If we were trying to prove a *single* case of environmentally mediated injury, we would probably not even try to apply cluster reasoning to prove the case in court, and therefore probably not to disprove it either. The cluster argument comes into play when there appear to be five or six victims – but we forget that this phenomenon could equally be seen as five or six *individual* victims, and argued on that basis.

Perhaps the underlying problem is that because of the environmental label we still perceive environmentally mediated injuries principally as public health problems – which reflects the start of this chapter. We are then drawn into arguing cases in a way that relies heavily on a medical perception of causation: epidemiology. If we were looking at a case of four assaults in one village, we would not ask the epidemiologist to provide the explanation, even if clusters of four assaults were a common phenomenon (and this could well be the case). We should therefore question more carefully why we would call in the epidemiologist to explain four environmentally mediated injuries. Is it that epidemiology can provide good answers, or that using epidemiology appeases our frustration at being unable currently to comprehend the causal links in environmental cases?

## The science–law time-lags

The time-lag between what science can do and what law must do is lucidly put by Pugh and Day in *Toxic Torts*:

> *A matter of real concern is whether scientific knowledge can keep up with some of the problems that science causes . . . In brain damage cases there are now highly sensitive scanning devices which will pick up damage which simply could not be seen with yesterday's technology. The fact that 10 years ago a mild to moderate traumatic brain damage claim sometimes failed for want of expert evidence to substantiate it whereas today the same claim would undoubtedly succeed is an eloquent reminder that the court should apply its common sense to causation issues as a jury would and not allow scientific theorising to dethrone fact. The use of common sense to fill the gaps where scientific understanding is incomplete has a perfectly respectable legal pedigree. If this is not robustly used the courts may leave the citizen to the mercy of 'junk' science or inept theory.*[11]

The scientist can only report in relation to the past; the law must protect us in the future.

The time-lag problem might appear to act only in one direction – science cannot provide definitive answers, so the courts make a common-sense judgement which takes account of the unknown. But the reverse is also the case: sometimes science does have knowledge but courts or committees cannot comprehend it.

Environmental cases can grind to a halt simply because courts cannot grasp the scientific evidence. The judge who was to try the Camelford aluminium case (Chapter 11) concluded that proving the causal link and severity of the injury would have been very problematic: 'If the case had been contested there would have been awesomely complex argument over how much [water] they consumed and you have been well advised to accept the offer.'[12] The comment is an interesting indictment of courts. Is complexity, however awesome, an acceptable reason why environmental victims should not achieve justice?

The problem goes deeper than understanding scientific technicalities, and enters the realms of philosophy. Reporting the not guilty verdict made in relation to leukaemia among children living near the Sellafield nuclear power station (UK), Tom Wilkie presents one such contradiction with great lucidity:

> *Radiation results from nuclear interactions that are governed by the laws of quantum mechanics. One of the least understood aspects of quantum physics is that there can be effects that do not have causes. It could be that the Sellafield cancers are an instance of this, and that yesterday's judgement demonstrated how the law of England has yet to catch up with the laws of quantum mechanics.*[13]

At the present time, if courts cannot comprehend what they do not know, the default mode is 'not guilty'.

But it would be wrong to leave this aspect of mismatch in the giddy realms of quantum mechanics. Imagine a court case in which a complainant in a less-wealthy nation claimed damages in relation to lead poisoning from the solder used to manufacture the cans of a regularly consumed brand of beans. The defendant might claim that a tin in its existing form is the safest option, because to use a plastic lining could expose customers to hormone-disrupting chemicals (Bisphenol-A) and that an aluminium can might precipitate dementia, even though the science in these two areas is far from conclusive. The judge might also be reminded that to rule that none of the options is acceptable would drastically curtail the means of food preservation and distribution in a country where nutrition was already poor to a level at which vitamin and micro-nutrient deficiencies could affect child development.

The judgement would not just be about a tin of beans, but about how a human population ensures its positive survival in the context of the modern world and its mass of uncertainties. This is already the underlying nature of many cases concerning environmentally mediated injury. Yet we entrust these decisions to courts running on much the same lines as they did two hundred years ago – an era before electricity, the splitting of the atom, synthetic chemicals and cars.

## Notes

1. L. Salter, *Mandated Science: Science and Scientists in the Making of Standards* (Kluwer: London, 1988), p. 123.

2. Walter J. Rogan *et al.* 'Congenital poisoning by polychlorinated biphenyls and their contaminants in Taiwan', *Science* (1988), **241**, 334.

3. EAJ, *Our Intensive Efforts to Overcome the Tragic History of Minamata Disease* (Environment Agency of Japan: Tokyo, 1992).

4. Nord, *Nordic Criteria for Reproductive Toxicity* (Nordic Council of Ministers: Copenhagen, 1992), pp. 23–4.

5. C. Pugh and M. Day, *Toxic Torts* (Cameron May: London, 1992), pp. 25, 51.

6. H.L.A. Hart and A.M. Honore, *Causation in the Law* (Oxford University Press: Oxford, 1985).

7. *R* v. *CICB ex parte P* 1993.

8. Martin Wainwright, 'Toxins ruled out in limb disorders', *Guardian*, 4 April 1995, p. 2.

9. Ruth Gilbert, '"Clusters" of anophthalmia in Britain', *British Medical Journal* (1993), **307**, 340–1.

10. Green Network. 'Boy born without eyes wins $4m court award', *Network News* (Colchester, UK) (1996), Summer, 8.

11. Pugh and Day, *op. cit.* (n. 5), pp. 25, 51.

12. Paul Brown, 'Water company offers £400,000 pollution payout', *Guardian*, 11 April 1994, p. 2.

13. Tom Wilkie, 'Probability stacked against radiation victims', *Independent*, 9 October 1993, p. 5.

# CHAPTER 13

# A New Ethical Consensus

Development within a justice system is usually preceded by an evolution of public ethics. Five areas are evident within which a new consensus must emerge, to address EMID and other environmentally mediated injuries.

Exactly what is an 'environmental victim'? The phrase is now in general use, but its meaning is unclear. More specifically, it is necessary to affirm the status of the unborn victim, because of the particular vulnerability of the embryo and foetus to EMID and other related hazards. Besides a clearer view of the victims, we also need to create a clearer view of the perpetrators: who is responsible and to what degree? Then, how do we link the two, victim and perpetrator: what is 'environmental causation'? Finally, how should we prove a causal link? In the context of common-sense decision-making in a court, should the burden of proof be adjusted to accommodate the problematic nature of environmentally mediated injury?

## The environmental victim

The term 'environmental victim' is coming into common usage, but its meaning is not clear.[1] A book called *Victims of the Environment*[2] only concerns natural disasters such as tornadoes and earthquakes, in which there are no apparent perpetrators. By contrast, in the headline 'Brain Damage Found in Victims of Bhopal Disaster'[3] the meaning is very different, as the environmental factors were not natural and there were culpable entities. In an editorial for India's environmental magazine *Down to Earth*, Anil Agarwal wrote of his experience of cancer: 'I was speaking not just as an environmental activist but also as an environmental victim.'[4] The phrase therefore arises naturally in discussion of contemporary environmental problems, but without sufficient precision.

Surprisingly, even 'environment' is rarely defined clearly in law or international declarations. Through usage, it is now generally taken to comprise four components: chemical, physical, microbiological and psycho-social. The importance of the last is in relation to corporate abuses of power which manipulate the other three components: for example, cigarette advertising aimed at children or developing countries.

The UN Declaration on victims . . . of abuse of power (1985) provides a basic framework for developing the concept of 'environmental victims'. It concerns 'persons who . . . have suffered harm, including . . . mental injury . . . through acts or omissions that do not yet constitute violations of national criminal laws but of internationally recognized norms relating to human rights'. The Declaration proposes that states should develop national and international legislation, and provide 'remedies to victims . . . [including] restitution and/or compensation, and necessary material, medical, psychological and social assistance and support'.

When formally defining 'environmental victims', it is helpful to exclude those more accurately described as 'environmental casualties', who suffer as a result of natural disasters. Implicit in the etymology of 'casualties' is the notion of *chance*, while the concept 'victims' embodies the idea of suffering caused by a *conscious* human act. Some circumstances that appear natural may, if analysed in greater depth, be a consequence of human acts. Those killed by recent floodings of the Yangtze River may have been victims of deforestation and soil erosion which precipitated the surge. Environmental suffering that has affected many generations, such as iodine deficiency, might not be seen as victimization until power relationships are examined – why are the communities that suffer iodine deficiency forced to live on land that cannot sustain human life properly?

Environmental law usually embodies the principle that the outcome of an act must have been 'reasonably foreseeable' for it to constitute an offence. But, so far, most environmental law relates to damage to the physical world, not human injury. If we are considering human injury as a specific outcome, it seems more appropriate to borrow from common law in relation to personal injury, as proposed at the end of Chapter 11. Here the principle is whether an act is deliberate or *reckless*, and reckless behaviour may not require foreseeing a *specific outcome*, simply that an act could, by its nature, be dangerous to others. The distinction is important. Many claims for compensation for environmentally mediated injury fail because the perpetrator maintains that it was impossible to foresee a specific outcome. For example, the dumping of a particular substance may be excused because it was not known, at the time, to be hazardous (the specific negative outcome was not 'foreseeable'). But, in the same circumstances, it might be claimed that to dump the substance was reckless because it was not proven safe. In the light of the inability of science to keep up with the problems it causes, this common-sense precautionary principle seems more in accord with human well-being. It is the tradition of common law on personal injury, not environmental protection, that has at its heart the direct well-being of humans.

The outcome of victimization is better described as 'injury' rather than 'suffering'. Injury, as an adverse health effect caused by environmental factors, is neatly defined by Christiani: 'any effect that results in altered structure or impaired function, or represents the beginnings of a sequence of events leading to altered structure or function'.[5] Implicit in the term injury is a relationship between two events (cause and effect) which culminate in tangible harm; suffering implies less acute general experiences which might be tolerated without actual injury. This distinction also addresses the idea, common now in poorer countries, that people must endure some environmental suffering for the benefits of economic development, such as road-building. This is an arguable trade-off, but in no justice system is it acceptable to trade off the infliction of human *injury* (or death) against economic benefit.

Intergenerational responsibility must be implicit in any conceptualization because of the time-latent nature of much environmental victimization. There also needs to be an assumption that both victims and perpetrators might be individuals or groups. And, as will be argued later in relation to causation, it is more appropriate to phrase a definition 'consequence of' rather than 'caused by'. 'Environmental victims' can therefore be defined as

> those of past, present or future generations who are injured as a
> consequence of change to the chemical, physical, microbiological
> or psycho-social environment, brought about by deliberate or
> reckless, individual or collective, human act or act of omission.

The etymology of 'victim' embodies 'sacrifice', and this underlying meaning provides a helpful insight. Environmental victims are often, in effect, sacrificed for the benefit of a more powerful entity. It is common for industrial polluters to argue that the environment of a few downstream or downwind individuals must be sacrificed for the greater good of improving national economies or providing employment. The US government now talks formally of toxic no-go areas as 'environmental sacrifice zones'. And, more chillingly, the local term for children downwind of US nuclear test sites in Nevada, who were born with birth impairments, is 'the sacrifice babies'.

## The unborn victim
One of the greatest inconsistencies running through the legislation discussed in Chapter 11 is the status of the unborn victim. Can a foetus be the victim of a criminal offence? Can a child sue because of injuries sustained in the womb? The questions are crucial. Uncertainty whether or not a right of

action existed in respect of an unborn child led to victims disabled by the drug thalidomide accepting an out-of-court settlement which is now seen as wholly inadequate.

The law is often very vague, and certainly not consistent on a global or even national level, so we need to piece together an understanding from disparate legal sources, and identify the ethical conflicts, which are mainly between a pregnant woman and her unborn child. The law can recognize a link between a woman consuming alcohol and the possibility of brain injury to a child resulting from her reckless driving, but does it recognize the link between a mother recklessly consuming alcohol and brain injury to her unborn child through foetal alcohol syndrome? The causal agent in the two circumstances is the same, the outcome of the injury for a child could be very similar, yet the law and our ethical agreement about its application is inconsistent between the two circumstances because the causal mechanisms are dissimilar.

One of the few attempts to clarify this question was the UK Law Commission report *Injuries to Unborn Children*.[6] Even in 1973, the authors were of the view that 'where a child is born with a disability which was caused by someone's fault occurring before birth, he should be entitled to recover damages from that person'. The report was prescient of issues such as drugs, irradiation and trauma. The early precedents come from North America and Australia. In 1933, the Supreme Court of Canada ruled very simply that 'a child, if born alive and viable, should be allowed to maintain an action in the courts for injuries wrongfully committed on its person while in the womb of its mother'.[7] An Australian judgement upheld this view in 1972, and is particularly interesting because no direct physical injury to the foetus, resulting from the motor accident, was proven. The cause of the intellectual injury to the child was seen as the trauma suffered by the mother.[8]

In the USA, before 1946, the unborn victim was rarely recognized, according to the Law Commission report, for two reasons:

● that the defendant could owe no duty of care to a person who was not in existence at the time of his (or her) 'negligent' act;

● that the difficulty of proving a causal connection between the act and the damage was too great and there was too much danger of fabricated claims.

Since that date, probably owing to the increased certainty of scientific proof, the USA has reached the point at which the courts of every US state hold, 'as a development of the common law and despite previous decisions to the contrary', that a child can recover damages for a pre-natal injury.

Paradoxically, the ambiguous status of the foetus can sometimes work to its *advantage*. Provision for workers' compensation in the USA abrogates the right of employees to sue employers for work-related harm, but this prohibition against tort probably does not extend to the foetus.

But doubts remain. Only a few US states acknowledge injury resulting from events happening *before* conception: for example, high body burdens of lead in a mother owing to previous employment, which then crosses to the foetus. This could be clarified by applying a 'man trap' test. If a farmer set a trap in 1990 which injured a 10-year-old child in 1995, the farmer would clearly be responsible for the injury. But what if the child were only 3 years old? Again there seems little doubt that the farmer would be seen as responsible – even though the victim had not been conceived at the time the trap was set.

The UK Congenital Disabilities Act 1976 aimed to uphold the rights of the unborn child, but did not give the child *independent* victim status. The child only has a right of action if the parent first suffers an actionable injury. Yet medical science tells us that an unborn child can be impaired by minute doses of chemicals, far too small to have any effect on an adult. With the curious exception of a mother who drives negligently, the unborn child is also not protected from its parents' wilful or careless behaviour, such as drugs abuse. Compensation is not payable if injury to the parent preceded conception and one or both parents knew of the risk of birth injury related to their job. It is unlikely that parents working in, for instance, a nuclear power station could prove that they did not know of the risk factor. Employers can therefore avoid liability to unborn children simply by telling employees that their work poses a reproductive hazard. A case will fail if the injury to the child resulted in part from parental negligence, or if parents consented to the hazard. This veiled use of the concept of 'contributory negligence' is bizarre: why is the victim status of unborn children diminished by the actions or knowledge of others over whom they can have no influence or control?

Compare this statutory denial of independent status with real-world circumstances. An embryo can now be created outside the womb, stored and implanted many years later into a woman's womb, not necessarily that of its biological mother. It has been proposed that stored embryos that have lost all connection with their biological parents should become wards of court to protect their interests. Technically, these 'limbo children' could be preserved for centuries, carrying an independent status well after their biological parents have died. In 1995, sperm taken from a father *after his death* was successfully used to fertilize his widow's ovum.[9] Under the Congenital Disabilities Act children born in this manner could be denied access to justice because of the actions of fathers who died before they were conceived. How would we link the status of the unborn child to the father or mother in the case of the rape and pregnancy of a New York woman who had been in a coma in hospital for ten years?

If current Japanese experiments are successful, the womb will soon be replaceable by a birth tank, and a child may never need any biological attachment to its mother. In these and countless other examples, the unborn child now has an independent organic and ethical status. Yet a statute intending to protect the unborn child makes it, in relation to environmental victimization, inseparable from its biological parents.

In 1992, a woman who kicked a pregnant neighbour in the stomach, causing fatal brain damage to the unborn child, was charged with manslaughter. This was the first case of its kind in the UK. An appeal ruling following a case in which a man stabbed his pregnant girlfriend affirmed that, if the unborn child died as a result, it would be possible to achieve a conviction for murder or manslaughter.[10] This raises many questions. What about an assault charge had the unborn child suffered non-fatal brain damage? Could a foetus be awarded compensation for injuries following a conviction for assault against its mother or itself? In the UK, an unborn child *could* be considered eligible for an award from the Criminal Injuries Compensation Board. A 1993 decision held: 'We accept that "personal injuries" is a term which can properly be applied to injuries occurring before birth and do not regard the precise stage at which injuries occurred as relevant to our decision.'[11] But would this include injuries resulting from something that happened before conception?

A UK Court of Appeal ruling in 1992 concluded that, although under English law an unborn child has no independent legal personality, courts will adopt the civil maxim that 'an unborn child shall be deemed to be born whenever its interests require it'. The 'child's best interests' caveat is interesting because it could address the conflict between giving the unborn child victim status, yet permitting abortion in the case of a potentially unwanted or unsupportable child or a seriously impaired foetus. In effect it proposes a moral view that death can be of secondary importance to injury. 'Child's best interests' does not resolve the moral conflicts, but the notion at least provides a basis on which to discuss them.

But there is a greater ethical question. How do we view abortion in relation to an unborn child who suffers serious impairment because of environmentally mediated injury – the foetus who has Down's syndrome because of radiation exposure from a government power station, for example? An abortion in this case, although perhaps in the child's best interests, might be seen as the execution of the victim in order to spare the perpetrator the cost of lifelong support. This is not a theoretical circumstance – it reflects the advice given to pregnant women by the USSR

A NEW ETHICAL CONSENSUS

government following the nuclear industry disaster in Chernobyl. China's Maternal and Infant Health Care Law 1994 'encouraging' (not just permitting) the abortion of impaired foetuses enshrines this dubious ethic in law. Unless the potential perpetrator can resolve this moral dilemma, the only possible ethical answer is to prevent the environmental exposure in the first place.

Conflicts between the interests of the unborn child and the mother are highly contentious. The 'right to work' provides a central area of debate. One outcome of the recognition of the unborn victim in the USA was workplace 'foetal protection policies'. But these were quickly used to discriminate against women as employees, rather than protect the unborn child, to the degree that employers insisted on the sterilization of women workers to prevent any possibility of compensation claims. Despite a Supreme Court ruling, which held that this interpretation violated the Pregnancy Discrimination Act, employers continue to ask women to sign waivers accepting responsibility for work-related risks.[12]

It is questionable that protection policies should relate so specifically to women. The exposure of men to reproductive hazards is, arguably, an equal threat to unborn children, but gender politics has culminated in a bias in reproductive science which means that the evidence is not yet available. Feminist academics have rightly challenged the inconsistencies, but have still not resolved the basic conflict that arises if a reproductively active person puts his or her right to work above the safety of the unborn child.

There are other child–mother conflicts. Pregnant American mothers who cause *in utero* injury because they use drugs are now being charged with 'distributing' drugs to their unborn babies. Could this mean that a child injured by drugs is entitled to compensation or damages from its mother? How does this precedent relate to alcohol abuse? Feminists have rightly argued for women to have control over their own bodies. Unfortunately, the discussion stops short at resolving the conflict between a woman's rights and those of her unborn child.

After birth, in the case of a conflict of interests between parent and child, the scales always tip in favour of the child. If the moral position concerning an unborn child is different, we must be clear why. It is an inescapable fact that a mother is the environment of her unborn child. If a mother accepts that her child has a right to an unhazardous environment after birth, it would be inconsistent for her to argue that the child did not have this right before birth, or to act in a way that jeopardized a healthy pre-natal environment.

The emerging precedents also raise questions concerning the day-to-day prevention of injury to an unborn child. A UK magistrates' court heard an application for bail from a pregnant woman, who was known to be abusing drugs and had attempted to kill herself by taking an overdose the day before the hearing. Could the magistrates have refused the woman unconditional bail on the grounds of 'preventing further offending' because of likely injury to her unborn child (i.e. an offence of assault or manslaughter)? In prison or bail hostel, the level of supervision might have prevented injury to the child. In some Canadian provinces, a pregnant woman abusing drugs can now lawfully be detained in a hospital for the protection of her unborn child. In South Carolina, pregnant women who refuse treatment for drugs abuse are being held in prison.

Cultural perspectives provide another dimension. Many traditional understandings – for example among the African Ashanti – do not accord children full human status until a naming ceremony one or two years *after* birth. A child who dies before this point may be buried in a cracked pot or with criminals, to symbolize its incomplete status. How, within such a context, do we argue for full recognition *before* birth?

Traditional beliefs appear to pose the problem, but with greater understanding perhaps they might also suggest answers. The Zulu saying 'Man is Man because of Man' proposes that we become human not only because we are born but because interaction with other human beings optimizes our human potential. This reflects the ethos of the naming ceremony, and would also accommodate necessary abortion and infanticide. But it might also be argued that any intellectual injury that impeded the optimizing interaction, even if sustained before birth, would be a serious concern.

There is one universally recognized traditional precedent for the prevention of birth impairments: incest taboos, which arose from the cumulative wisdom that babies born from consanguineous relationships were frequently intellectually impaired. There is also one centuries-old precedent that protects the unborn child and upholds its independent status, common to traditional law and sophisticated legislative codes alike: the death penalty can always be deferred for a woman if she is pregnant.

## Responsibility

Turning from victims to the recognition of perpetrators, environmentally mediated injury raises two problems. First, we need to develop a consensus about responsibility which recognizes the involvement of those who may carry some, but not total, responsibility for an act of victimization. Second, there is a need to recognize large perpetrator groups such as motorists, even if to propose 'guilt' in such circumstances is not a viable idea. Driving a car may not be seen as a deliberate act of poisoning, and it may not even poison, but the driver still carries some responsibility for the overall toxic soup which poses a 'violent' threat of environmentally mediated injury.

There are a few instances of innovative approaches to these problems. In terms of law, one of the more interesting followed the Union Carbide poisoning at Bhopal. In 1991, the Indian government enacted legislation requiring hazardous industries to take out special public liability insurance. This addresses the difficulty of identifying the individual perpetrators of corporate victimization, and might achieve quicker payment. Ethically this approach has advantages, because the law disperses the cost of compensation among those who benefit from taking the risks associated with hazardous industries – specifically those controlling and working for the factories, but also those who benefit through buying the resultant products. But the familiar spatial inconsistencies still pertain – central or state government-owned industries may be exempted under the Indian legislation, the informal sector is not covered, and therefore many of the most hazardous processes are excluded. It is also possible that such insurance schemes could encourage companies to take even greater risks. Why not, if you may not have to finance the consequences? Perhaps most importantly, the scheme does not embody the principle of deterrence.

From a theoretical perspective, in a discussion of the failings of civil law in relation to radiological risks, Christopher Miller proposes an 'environmental tax' on hazardous industries which would generally fund the public services that potentially have to provide support for environmental victims.[13] Although appealing for its simplicity, again this could decrease the incentive to avoid risks, and there is no deterrent. And from an ethical perspective, the idea that hazardous industries could buy off the public in this manner is very questionable.

Another approach is to rethink the *levels* of responsibility. Currently, levels are reflected in the rather arbitrary criminal–civil distinction, reflecting public–personal interest. Environmentally mediated injury clouds this traditional divide. All too often a civil claim provides the only route of redress in relation to, for example, radiation exposure from a power station. Yet surely this circumstance would embody a public interest factor at least equal to a parking ticket, which is a criminal matter. We need to develop levels that go across the traditional criminal–civil divide. From the emerging ethical debate it is possible to propose three levels of responsibility:

- *blame*, which entails conscious guilt, embracing deliberate and reckless acts or omissions by individuals;

- the *liability* of individuals or organizations answerable for a failure, in relation to reckless and negligent acts for which it would be unreasonable or impossible to attribute direct blame to individuals;

● *implication* of those whose involvement is not plainly expressed, but who intended to benefit from circumstances related to victimization.

It is likely that most forms of environmental victimization would entail responsibility at all levels. For example, a manager of a plastics factory may be to *blame* for a deliberate release of a toxin. The whole company might be considered *liable*, through not operating systems to prevent individual misdeeds. Those who intended to benefit from the production of the plastics, such as by buying plastic products, holding shares in the company or working in the factory, are *implicated* and must carry some responsibility. They should therefore compensate the general community in which victims live through a future levy on the product or wages.

This last category defines a new class of responsibility, to some extent reflecting Miller's 'environmental tax'. But its application is in relation to specific acts of victimization, and it covers the large, politically problematic perpetrator groups such as motorists. It would, for example, be administratively very easy to increase motor tax and direct the revenue to state health services, following cases such as that brought under the Indian Constitution, which found the government guilty of not controlling vehicle pollution.

The implicating factor is *intended benefit* ('intended' because it should be no defence that investment in a polluting factory showed no financial gain). Financial agents, such as banks, that support polluting industries are clearly implicated in the consequences of public poisoning, and there is an emerging moral consensus that this should be so. Implication through benefit also overrides the disclaimer by transnational companies that they do not formally own the hazardous industries in other countries. If they benefit through *any* form of commercial relationship, that is sufficient to view them as implicated in any related environmental victimization.

Implication preserves the principle of deterrence. But more importantly, the construct also rewards those who make an effort to ensure that they are not implicated: for example, those who do not buy products that cannot be manufactured or disposed of without creating toxins, those who refuse to work for companies that make profits by creating environmentally mediated hazards and those who only invest through ethically responsible banks.

One of the new tactics employed by polluting industries is to jump *directly* from a policy of outright denial to one of generous remediation. This neatly misses out the important stage in the middle – accepting responsibility. The approach of Shell concerning environmental degradation in the Niger delta, in 1996, demonstrated this approach. Remediation appeases victims and leads activists to believe that they have won a victory. In the long term the victimizer appears as the defender of environmental standards, and it is conveniently forgotten who caused the problem in the first place.

The purpose of any criminal justice system is to ensure that this form of buy-off does not happen, because there is an overriding public interest. The reckless driver who kills a child cannot simply close the matter by writing a generous cheque to the mother. Criminal justice maintains that there is a matter of public interest in addition to compensation, and the driver must answer to the state and acknowledge responsibility. Extending the perception of responsibility in relation to environmental victimization, to include implication, also extends the degree to which we can hold *all* those involved in victimization morally and then if necessary legally accountable for their behaviour.

## What is environmental causation?

Once we can define victims and agree the responsibility of perpetrators, the next stage is the link between the two – causation. It is convenient for an activist to talk of problems as 'environmentally caused', but a cause in relation to the above definition of 'environmental victim' is human interaction with the environment, not the environment itself (hence 'environmentally mediated'). The understanding of causation therefore requires greater clarity.

First, there is a conceptual legacy within law that must be questioned: the requirement that cause and effect must be adjacent. The law is usually framed in terms such as '*proximate* cause', '*immediate* violence' or 'a *continuing, operating* and substantial cause', reflecting the rule of criminal jurisprudence *causa proxima non remote spectatur*. Existing law has therefore been weak at conceptualizing the indirect nature of environmental victimization.

But, as outlined in Chapter 11, even the traditional perception of personal injury is now being stretched to accommodate new circumstances such as the spreading of HIV/AIDS infection, or the violent use of communications systems. Causal understandings of 'interjacency' are needed – embracing space, time and the multiplicity and interaction of causes and effects, and reflecting the 'creeping disasters' or, in UNICEF terms, 'slow emergencies' which now threaten human safety. Court judgements provide one source of evolving concepts, such as that of 'major contributory cause', which accepts that partial responsibility can mean full liability. It is now common for politicians to calm public concern by claiming that 'there is no immediate danger' from a new hazard. What do they mean: in the next ten minutes or the next ten years? These immediacy caveats need to be constantly challenged.

Another approach to the problem can derive from the importance of how the causal question is phrased. This is raised by Hart and Honore,[14] who cite a judge who considered the form 'Did the injury cause X?' inferior to 'Did X result from the injury?', and argue that their own preferred form is 'Was X the consequence of Y?', rather than 'Was Y the cause of X?'. This proposal was not made in relation to environmentally mediated injury, and might appear pedantic, but curiously when applied to real-life environmental problems it makes great sense. For example, if a toxic release degraded farmland, leading to malnutrition, and then to a high incidence of disability in the local population, it is easy to argue that the toxic release did not 'cause the disability' – the direct cause was malnutrition. It is less easy to argue that the disability was 'not a consequence' of the release.

How should environmental causation be defined in legal or quasi-legal terms? One approach is the recognition of environmentally mediated causation as the *presence* or *absence* of environmental factors, each of these embracing the standard distinction in criminal and civil laws defining offences, and therefore victimization, as stemming from human *acts* or *omissions*. Broadly, environmental causation would then fall into four groups, which are shown in Figure 13.1. Specific instances of victimization may well fit within more than one of these four categories, or may fit better in a different category at different periods over a long time scale (i.e. in the case of 'creeping disasters').

|  | **Act** | **Omission** |
|---|---|---|
| **Presence** of environmental agent | E.g. the *presence* of methyl isocyanate caused by an *act* of polluting and poisoning (Union Carbide, Bhopal) | E.g. the *presence* of excess lead in water supplies caused by an *omission* of the duty to provide safe drinking water |
| **Absence** of environmental agent | E.g. the *absence* of food and micro-nutrients, leading to malnutrition and brain injury, resulting from land degradation caused by the *act* of dumping toxic waste | E.g. the *absence* of iodine caused by an *omission* to iodize salt in accordance with the law (India) |

**Figure 13.1** A model of environmental causation.

The model is not hypothetical. Although scattered, laws and judgements already exist which acknowledge these four forms of environmentally mediated causation. For example, legislation redresses the *absence* of iodine in the environment by a statutory requirement that iodine is included in salt. Victimization, if iodine is not added to salt, therefore results from an *omission*. A UK Court of Appeal ruling in 1995 found that 'running a sewerage system in an unmaintained state is sufficient to entitle a jury to find the party responsible for the system guilty of causing pollution . . . failure implied an omission'.[15] This provides an instance of *presence/omission*. A definition emerges from this model, that environmental causation involves:

> a presence or absence of chemical, physical, micro-biological, or psycho-social environmental factors, resulting from individual or collective human act or omission, over any time-scale, of which the consequence is human injury.

## Burden of proof

If we have agreed what constitutes environmental causation, the next stage is to *prove* causal links – usually 'beyond reasonable doubt' in criminal cases and 'on the balance of probabilities' in civil law (did something 'more likely than not' cause a particular outcome). This is a fraught aspect of environmental victimization. In *No Immediate Danger*, Rosalie Bertell explained how the US nuclear industry's claim that reactors were safe arose from the difficulty of proving individual cases rather than the weight of scientific knowledge about the hazard. In relation to proof, the Atomic Energy Commission (AEC) held absolute power over the rules and procedure within which its own activities would be judged. Quoting the AEC's rules, Bertell concluded:

> *Not only is the industry assumed 'innocent' until proven guilty beyond a shadow of doubt (every other possible cause must be proven not responsible), but it is admitted that the proof required is 'not always attainable'. In fact, using ordinary vital statistics as collected in the USA and most other places, it can never be proven . . . it is impossible to 'satisfactorily eliminate every other factor known to influence the birth or death trait in contention'. Inadequate government record-keeping, plus the AEC philosophy, produces a vicious circle in which the victim is unable to 'prove' damage by the AEC rules.*[16]

Nowhere outside the field of environmentally mediated impacts are potential perpetrators permitted to dictate and control the rules concerning burden of proof in relation to personal injury in this manner.

Currently, in environmental cases the victim usually must prove that

● an injury was suffered;

● the environmental agent can cause the injury;

● the environmental agent was released;

- the victim was exposed (spatial evidence, temporal evidence, medical evidence);

- the known level of exposure could cause the injury;

- there was no other cause including 'natural' (medical evidence, epidemiological evidence).

Because complexity usually makes this burden of proof an impossibility, there is a trend towards accepting less strict standards. Outside the environmental sphere, rape cases provide a parallel. The evidence of the victim alone is being given increasing weight because the nature of the offence renders the more usual modes of proof unavailable.

It is arguable that, if a primary environmental offence has been committed, the offender should be put in the position of having to disprove secondary consequences, including injury. There is a precedent from recent British legislation concerning aggravated vehicle-taking. If the victim claims that damage has been done to a stolen vehicle by the thief, it is for the perpetrator to prove otherwise. This 'guilty until proven innocent' approach is considered reasonable because the primary offence of taking the vehicle denies the victim the possibility of proving the secondary offences. Another intriguing precedent comes from Canada, which, although unrelated to environmental causation, addresses multiple causation. The case concerned a man who was injured by a shot from one of two hunters who both fired carelessly in his direction at the same moment. The court accepted that as both hunters had been reckless, and that the outcome made it impossible for the victim to identify the perpetrator, the burden should be put on the hunters to prove their innocence.[17]

Recent environmental legislation from Germany also embodies this principle.[18] There is a presumption of causation if the environmental agents concerned are inclined to cause the injury – the victim need only prove the propensity of the agent to cause an effect. Only if the defendant can prove that he or she acted entirely within the law and other regulations does the victim take on the full burden of proof.

Embracing this approach, and other arguments in Part V, an alternative model for the burden of proof might be framed as follows.

*The victim (or state) must prove that:*

- an actual injury, or the circumstances of a potential injury, occurred;

- the injury can be a consequence of the presence (or absence) of the environmental agent;

- there was a release (or culpable absence) of the environmental agent.

*If so, the defendants are held responsible (to blame, liable or implicated; see p. 227) unless they can prove that:*

- the victim was not exposed to (or denied) the agent (spatial evidence, temporal evidence, medical evidence);

- the injury could not be a consequence of the exposure (or absence);

- there was another wholly responsible cause (medical evidence, epidemiological evidence if appropriate).

In the light of the current burden of proof placed upon environmental victims, it is illuminating to note circumstances in which politicians seem able instantly to modify the situation. When the US Congress was asked to set up a disability compensation scheme for Gulf War veterans and their offspring, following claims of a high incidence of health problems and birth impairments, the chairman of the Senate Banking Committee asked that claims be met, 'regardless of the ability to arrive at a definitive diagnosis'.[19] A little later, the Secretary for Veterans Affairs went even further and told a Congressional panel:

> *Their problems cannot be made to fit our solutions, so we must change the solutions . . . We don't know what is wrong with them, but we do know there is a physical or organic base to their problems, and we believe that the government should respond to their needs . . . we are going to give our veterans the benefit of the doubt. It will take time to resolve these scientific questions. In the mean time our veterans are still sick — so it is the right thing to do to move forward by providing them with compensation for their undiagnosed problems.*[20]

Environmentally mediated injury, suffered in relation to the defence of American interests, suddenly demanded a significant reduction of the burden of proof. So why was the legislation that increased the burden of proof in relation to the victims of nuclear testing in Nevada not repealed immediately (Chapters 6 and 11)? Situation ethics has its place, but its purpose is to achieve consistency through difference, not inconsistency through a difference created by political expediency.

## Principles for the prevention and redress of environmentally mediated injury

To argue for consistency is to argue not for sameness, but for difference that permits equity. For example, a consistent punishment policy for all those who steal $50 is not that they all receive the same sentence. A consistent response might range from prison for repeat offenders or for a police officer who abuses a position of trust and steals from a suspect, to an absolute discharge for someone who steals in order to eat, or treatment for an individual with mental health problems.

The key points are not complicated, and can be proposed as a set of principles.

*In relation to law, regulation, the achievement of justice, research methods or implementation*

1 There should be *no spatial inconsistencies*: between and across nations, workplaces, public places and domestic settings. Caveats such as 'proximate' should never prevent reasonable redress or protection.

2 There should be *no temporal inconsistencies*: intergenerational and time-latent effects should not be excluded, there should be no time limits on compensation claims for personal injury and cases should be resolved without unreasonable delay. Caveats such as 'immediate' should never prevent redress or protection.

3 There should be no *human inconsistencies*: the unborn child should have full independent victim status, and variation in relation to gender should only be on the basis of indisputable difference. 'Safe levels' should be constructed in relation to the *most* vulnerable human, in any discrepancy the precautionary principle should be applied by accepting the level that affords the greatest protection, and safe levels based on the 'average human' construct should not be permitted as a defence.

*Within and across spatial, temporal and human consistency*

1 Special legislation should *never diminish general rights* established within basic law, common law, human rights agreements or the prevailing view of natural justice.

2 Following any *prima facie* environmentally mediated hazard, or any act or omission by the perpetrator that increases the difficulty of evidencing causal relationships, the *burden of proof* should be on perpetrators to establish that the consequences of the hazard did not cause, or threaten, injury.

3 *Responsibility* should be recognized in terms of blame, liability and implication through intended benefit.

If framed in the form of a human right, the aim of a new ethical understanding in relation to EMID could be expressed very simply as upholding, for individuals and communities,

A right to the protection of innate intellectual potential against environmentally mediated hazards.

## Notes

1. Christopher Williams, 'An environmental victimology', *Social Justice* (1996), **23**(4), 16–40.

2. Peter H. Rossi *et al.*, *Victims of the Environment: Loss from Natural Hazards in the United States* (Plenum Press: New York, 1983).

3. BMJ, 'Brain damage found in victims of Bhopal disaster', *British Medical Journal* (1994), **309**, 359.

4. Anil Agarwal, 'Editorial', *Down to Earth*, 31 December 1996, p. 4.

5. E. Chivian *et al.*, *Critical Condition: Human Health and the Environment* (MIT Press: Cambridge, MA, 1993), p. 15.

6. Law Commission, *Injuries to Unborn Children*, working paper no. 47 (The Law Commission: London, 1973).

7. *Montreal Tramways* v. *Leveille* 4 DLR 337.

8. *Watt* v. *Rama* 1972.

9. Jonathan Freedland, 'Sperm extracted from corpse in world first', *Guardian*, 21 January 1995, p. 12.

10. Clare Dyer, 'Judge wrong over "killing" of baby', *Guardian*, 25 November 1995, p. 7.

11. *R* v. *CICB ex parte* P 1993.

12. Sally J. Kenney, *For Whose Protection? Reproductive Hazards and Exclusionary Policies in the United States and Britain* (University of Michigan Press: Ann Arbor, 1992).

13. C.E. Miller, 'Radiological risks and civil liability', *Journal of Environmental Law* (1989), **1**(1), 22–4.

14. H.L.A. Hart and A.M. Honore, *Causation in the Law* (Oxford University Press: Oxford, 1985), pp. 87, 135.

15. Ying Hui Tan, 'Unmaintained sewage system caused pollution', *Independent*, 31 January 1995, p. 11.

16. Rosalie Bertell, *No Immediate Danger* (London: Women's Press, 1985).

17. *Cook* v. *Lewis* [1952] 1 DLR 1.

18. Umwelthaftungsgesetz-UmweltHG, 1991. Section 6[I]; 6[II].

19. S. Tisdall, 'Iraq "used US biotoxins in Gulf war"', *Guardian*, 11 February 1994, p. 13.

20. Martin Walker, 'US to compensate Gulf war veterans', *Guardian*, 10 June 1994, p. 10.

# CHAPTER 14

# The Challenges to Human Intelligence

Does the small-scale evidence of EMID indicate something bigger? The answer to the central question of *Terminus Brain* does not come from simply counting the pieces of the jigsaw puzzle, not least because many pieces are missing. It emerges from how those pieces are fitted together and, most importantly, what that incomplete image then tells us about the gaps. Not everyone in the world suffers from EMID, but everyone is now part of a local or regional community that suffers its consequences.

The basic EMID paradigm reminds that there are no comprehensive assessments of the problem (Figure 1.1). Single-substance science creates narrow perceptions of environmental impacts on the brain.[1] No statistic adds together the degree of intellectual decline arising from a range of different environmental neurotoxins, and there are no statistical projections that embrace time-latency – the cumulative and intergenerational effects. Nowhere is there mention of the combined outcomes of *absence*-EMID and *presence*-EMID. *Synergistic* effects could be the most significant dynamic, but there has been no attempt to find out.[2] Research tends to investigate the obvious 'clinical' outcomes such as Down's syndrome, which gives the impression of an unfortunate but limited problem, but few studies go further and assess the more widespread 'sub-clinical' consequences of the same causal factor.[3] All forms of adverse environmental change may create health impacts leading to the over-use of medical drugs and other techniques that can cause *iatrogenic* brain impairment, but we have no idea of the level of impact on intellectual resources.[4]

At one level, the answer to the *Terminus Brain* question is that prevailing conceptualizations, current techniques and resultant statistics demonstrate only the *minimum* impact of EMID. Although a few specific studies exaggerate their case, it is hard to find any argument about the broader picture that overstates the problem.

But at another level, the 'something bigger' goes beyond an assessment of scale. The most significant gaps in the jigsaw concern the future. What are the implications of EMID in relation to individual and human survival in the long and medium term, and what are the immediate challenges?

## The long term

Looking into the future, over millennia, EMID gives rise to two significant uncertainties about positive human survival.

First is the conflict between human self-interest and ecological self-interest. Intellectual decline is inconvenient for individuals and detrimental for communities – but in the long term potentially good news for the environment. For humans, EMID is the result of environmental problems; for the ecosystem it appears to be a solution to those problems.[5] Our dysfunctional behaviour towards our environment has put a premium on the brain's downward mobility, from the long-term eco-perspective.

We are unlikely to discover the full potential of eco-intelligence to redress human behaviour until it is too late. But we might at least consider questions that give rise to the uncertainty. For example, when we excessively contaminate our environment with a toxin such as lead, the ecosystem does not ultimately opt to provide an effective sink that disposes of, or mechanism that converts, this substance in a manner that inherently protects our intelligence. Eco-mechanisms probably could adapt to render such a toxin completely harmless to us: 'environmentally mediated' is not synonymous with threat. So why not?

Is it perhaps because such substances are function-disrupting across a spectrum of biological eco-entities – not just our brain – so there needs to be an overarching ecological defence strategy? Instead of ultimately protecting the human brain, the ecosystem maintains substances such as lead in a form that could eventually restrict the ability and behaviour of the eco-entity that creates the function-disrupting threat in the first place – that brain. Are we quite certain that this is not a rational response from an ecosystem that is in some manner intelligent?

One challenge for our intelligence, therefore, is to work out the risk associated with our current environmental behaviour, in the context of our ignorance as to whether the ecosystem could act against us and change that behaviour. Perhaps ecological intelligence can detect and control aspects of human intelligence – perhaps it cannot. But if it could it probably would, and we don't know that it can't.

The second uncertainty is that we might create environmental conditions that lead to regressive brain evolution in some populations.[6] A favourable environment led to progressive evolution – unfavourable environments could perhaps lead to regression. The uncertainty is that we do not know the size of environmental impact required to precipitate degenerative spirals.

This raises related considerations. One is that the evolutionary pattern of humans now presents our brain as particularly susceptible to environmental insults. We are born more prematurely than other species, so the young brain is very fragile in infancy. Our brain is more complex than that of other species, and complex organisms tend to be less robust, in relation to toxic insult and in needing a very specific and balanced nutritional intake. We are high up the food chain, and therefore environmental toxins are at their greatest concentrations when they reach us.[7] Add to this list the fact that personal survival is in the context of an exceptionally demanding social environment,[8] and consequently any slight impairment of intellectual function has a disproportionate impact on our day-to-day existence.

In the ecological context, high intelligence seems symbiotic with a high vulnerability of its organic host. If in addition extreme intelligence is linked with extreme ecologically dysfunctional behaviour, the intelligence–vulnerability symbiosis presents an automatic mechanism to correct the dysfunction.

The current environmental threat to our brain also seems unique in the history of human evolution. EMID is a new experiment. But evolutionary perspectives can be overstated. The brain's survival in a different human-made environment may not be inherently threatened. The intellectual challenge is simply to keep in mind, and calculate the risk associated with, a new circumstance.

The human brain developed to its current favourable condition within an environment in a 'natural' state. On the whole, during the period of human existence, this seems to have changed only very slowly over millions of years. Our brain is not the product of the human-created environment that is rapidly taking over, which now changes radically within single generations. The main threat to the brain may come less from specific chemical changes within its environment, and more from an increased instability and unpredictability within that chemical soup.

The next consideration is from the evolutionary theorists, who conclude that the biological evolution of the human brain has already reached a pinnacle,[9] irrespective of EMID. Our current highly intelligent brain may be just a biological aberration – an accident that has given rise to a behavioural extreme that will inevitably turn back towards the mean at some point. Could EMID tip the scales? Whatever the reality, our intelligence is obviously a fragile product of a very special set of evolutionary circumstances, and that fact itself should engender caution.

A broader consideration arises from viewing the human brain as just another part of the overall ecosystem. Our brain creates the environmental threat that it now poses to itself, and there seems to be no other piece of organic matter in the ecosystem that behaves like this. Eco-entities are commonly at risk through competition from other parts of the ecosystem, but nothing except the human brain is at direct risk from itself. Contrary to popular belief, even lemmings do *not* 'behave like lemmings'. This unique behaviour surely makes our brain uniquely vulnerable.

Certain plants produce natural pesticides as part of their survival mechanism – the tobacco plant is an example. If ecologists discovered a plant of this type, but its toxic output created a local environment that then threatened to poison and disrupt the functioning of that same species, or destroy the local micro-nutrients vital for its survival, they would be astonished. They would observe and monitor the self-imposed demise of the species with great interest, and there might even be a campaign group arguing for human intervention. This scenario reflects the current circumstance of the human brain as an eco-entity, yet we are neither astounded nor even much interested – and there is no higher intelligence to campaign on our behalf.

## Why does our brain now knowingly create environmentally mediated self-threats?

This surely must be one of the most intriguing and important questions of our era: the age of self-injury.

Our intellectual abilities drive the dynamics of EMID, principally in relation to energy creation and information processing.[10] And our intellectual shortcomings play a part, not least our seeming inability to perceive the consequences of human behaviour when magnified by large populations. It is very evident that humans also have a behaviour trait that underpins our self-destructive relationship with our environment, which, for want of a better term, can be called pertinacity.[11]

If we look at pertinacity in the context of human evolution, EMID may signify an inherent flaw in the way in which our species has reached its pre-eminence. An organism that is (in the words of the *OED* definition of pertinacious) 'persistent and stubborn in holding to its own opinion or design' may well have had an evolutionary advantage – but only up to a point. Pertinacious behaviour may have permitted human supremacy in the context of a survival of the fittest. But it may also be a form of intelligence that is not infinitely fit to survive.

That the human brain now *knowingly* creates this environmental self-threat leads inevitably to the debate about human consciousness. If the brain is, as Francis Crick maintains, 'nothing but a pack of neurons',[12] how do we explain this ecologically unique self-threat? No other bits of biomass seem to behave in this way. Yet even if the human brain does have a distinctive form of non-organic consciousness, the same question can be asked, but with greater incredulity.

Perhaps instead of fuelling a circular argument, the EMID self-threat might prompt an alternative way to conceptualize human consciousness. So far, the search has been based on the fast-increasing knowledge of the biology of the brain and the nature of mind. The quest has been largely inward-looking.

Crick may well be right to argue that we should understand consciousness principally in terms of neurons,[13] but why stop there with the context of a biological explanation? Rather than trying to identify consciousness just within the context of the human brain, and in relation to the higher orders of animals (the phylogenetic scale), we could also seek to understand its identity within the context of the whole ecosystem.

The consciousness theorists cannot make an absolute divide between human and animal consciousness. And even the distinction between plants and animals may not be as clear-cut as we think. For instance, new understandings of brown algae propose that these are plant–animal hybrids.[14] Remember then the *Photobacterium ficheri*, those quorum-sensing microbes that recognize when their population grows above a certain point and respond by producing more light.[15] Arguably, by some definitions, quorum-sensing is conscious behaviour.

It sometimes seems that the only purpose of enquiry into human intelligence and consciousness is to boost the human ego and affirm our belief in human difference and therefore supremacy. Instead of asking what is so distinct and separate about human consciousness and its biological host our brain, we should perhaps ask: what does it have in common with, and how is it still related to, the eco-intelligence that gave birth to human intelligence? Within this context, the nature of our collective human intelligence, which currently seems to misinform and misdirect our individual intelligence so radically, might become more evident. And through that we might understand better why, standing distinct from all other eco-entities, the human brain is now at risk from itself.

## The medium term: greater divides

Looking forward over millennia can seem an irrelevance in the light of what is a here-and-now problem. What is the medium-term scenario: what might happen over the next two hundred years? Might we witness a general decline in human intelligence?

It is indisputable that in wealthy communities, over the past century, improved nutrition, health, education and workplace safety have permitted incremental improvements in intellectual resources, which, combined with sophisticated management of those resources, have led to astonishing human achievements. Many of the environmental hazards of modernity are also challenging in a manner that is intellectually stimulating. Coping with traffic – driving or crossing busy roads daily – probably develops forms of perception that have only recently been awakened in the human brain. It is claimed that in the UK, USA, Japan and other rich countries national IQ has *increased* in the past fifty years by around 5 to 10 points[16] – although that does not mean that EMID has had no impact in those countries.

This leads to a conclusion about the medium term that is more subtle than a simple progression *or* regression model. What we will probably witness is not a general intellectual decline, but a furthering of the division between an elite generally within rich communities, and a disadvantaged majority generally within poorer communities. This is not just a futuristic scenario. To some extent we have already arrived there, but we dress up the divide in sound bites such as 'lack of education', which are politically more acceptable than admitting the degree to which the human brain is not responding to the adverse environmental challenges that it now poses itself.

Meritocracy and social differentiation are not new, but EMID creates a novel dynamic. Until now, meritocratic social divides have generally arisen because of the *upward* extension of intellectual potential – better health, nutrition and education have produced new cadres of intellectual elites. EMID furthers the divide by *downward* extension. If the two operate simultaneously the result can only be even greater divides.

Add to this the demographic factor. Those nations generally creating differentiation through upward extension are also the nations where birth rates are static or, in the case of Japan, declining. Birth rates are generally higher in poor communities than in rich, and the poor are the greater percentage of the world's population. Downward extension is likely to affect more people, creating a drag on our global intellectual resource.

In the context of a century or two, the conundrum therefore is that the agents of both positive and adverse intellectual development are often the same: transport, medicine, power-generation, building construction. If the modern environmental challenge is potentially both good and bad, how do we sort out which is which to inform an overarching policy? There are few golden rules, but Florence Nightingale's advice to nurses is a good guide: 'The *first* duty is to do no harm.' *After* that has been achieved we can experiment with permitting the challenges that might lead to positive change.

## The immediate challenge: acceptance

It seems very unlikely that the modernity dynamics that drive the causes of EMID will be reversed in the immediate future. The challenge to our intelligence to find eventual solutions is probably not beyond our capabilities; many people will find the search stimulating and rewarding, and doubtless many careers will be made in the process. But the immediate challenge facing us is far less glamorous, and therefore in many ways more difficult. Like it or not, in the near future the world will have increased numbers of people who suffer EMID in varying degrees of severity. The challenge is not just one of providing adequate public services, although that will be formidable; it is the full social *acceptance* of people who suffer intellectual decline.

Except in a few settings, people with intellectual disabilities are commonly ostracized, hidden, abused and forgotten.[17] Even people who just appear a little slow are the butt of jokes and subtle forms of alienation which are an accepted norm in every part of the world. Attitudes towards dementia are especially problematic. For a young child with an intellectual disability there does at least seem some hope of development, which will reward those who provide support. For older people no such motivation arises.

Changes must start within the professions. Currently, specialization in intellectual disability within medicine is not seen as prestigious. The field attracts the remarkable few who do not clamour for the fame and fortune associated with more glamorous forms of medicine. For medics, research about the prevention of disability usually assumes greater importance than that about providing effective care. This will need to change. Peripheral areas of social work – for example, supporting people with intellectual disabilities to raise families – will need to assume far greater importance in the future. Schoolteachers will certainly have to develop more constructive attitudes and strategies in relation to under-achievement and behaviour difficulties among their pupils.[18]

Acceptance will need to go beyond the caring professions, and enter the whole structure of democratic governance. In the UK or North America many people with significant intellectual disabilities will now vote at national and local elections. With the help of care workers their choices will be informed by an awareness of the basic policies of all candidates, and they might have met some of the candidates. Their choice may well be better informed than that of some other citizens in the same countries. By contrast, in countries such as India, millions of intelligent but often illiterate people will vote for the person whom they are told, or bribed, to vote for. An intelligent democracy need not be dependent solely on high individual intelligence across all citizens, but on acceptance of the intellectual resource as it is, and the provision of appropriate help.

If we cannot change attitudes in a way that will lead to the unconditional acceptance of all human beings irrespective of their intellectual status, we will create forms of social division that, even in its wildest dreams, the nineteenth-century eugenics movement could not have imagined. The key is how we value 'other' human beings, which stems from how we see them, which comes from knowing them as individual people, not just as statistics.

## Muddling through

In a world labelled postmodern, we are to believe that there are now no absolute truths. It seems correct that grand theories and ideologies have served us no better, and sometimes considerably worse, than muddling through with *ad hoc* responsive governance and patchwork policy. But in the context of the overwhelming nature of global problems, there does still seem to be one principle worth preserving. Things will probably be better for us all if our collective intellectual resources are maintained and managed at a functional level.

Education, the great saviour of the twentieth century, has not managed to reach this goal. Even in its liberationist form, organized education generally achieves little more than letting some people survive well at the expense of others. It rarely has an *equitable* impact on intellectual resources and individual survival across whole communities.

From the evidence of the education debate of the past fifty years, few would claim that formal or non-formal school systems have proven that they can have the desired universal impact. But the universal education experiment *has* demonstrated a remarkable consensus, which, in the context of human history, is relatively new. Whatever the political, religious or academic ideology – communism, capitalism, Catholicism, Confucianism – all parts of the spectrum have agreed that optimizing intellectual resources is important, and that *this cannot be left to chance in the modern world*.

In the contemporary context, to see schooling as the main route to achieving this end is probably now a mistake. That was a twentieth-century idea, which can now only be part of a broader strategy. Globally, the fundamental aim should be to prevent adverse impacts on intellectual potential. When that has been addressed – when we 'do no harm' – education can put the icing on the cake.

Education ministries, especially in the less wealthy regions, might well be restructured as ministries of intellectual resources, embracing the spectrum of relevant concerns, from intellectual disability (which is not really a matter for health ministries) to universities, from work training for young people of modest abilities to appropriate educational provision for elderly people with dementia; and, most importantly, implementing comprehensive strategies for preventing and mitigating EMID. For example, with high-tech distance-learning assuming a greater importance in less wealthy regions, ensuring the optimum intellectual receptivity of target communities is essential. Maintaining both the satellite dish *and* the micro-nutrient status of communities is a key to effective distance-learning in rural India.

Education faculties could reflect this change and broaden from a narrow concern with schools to become faculties of intellectual development. Research might make links between formal education, life-long learning, parenting, EMID and appropriate responses to the intellectual resource of a community *as it exists*: the ability of people of low intelligence to participate in democratic processes, for example. Schools might then progress from being exam factories to become fully integrated health–welfare–education child development centres – and the hub of activities that optimize the intellectual potential of the whole local community.

Street children who learn to beg by saying 'please' fare better than the ones who just tug at your sleeve. They enhance their survival through their intelligence, not in the academic meaning but through what people in northern England would call 'nous' – gumption or common sense. At this level of human survival, education finds it hard to know what to teach, yet human beings can often work out what to learn, if they have a functional ability to learn. There are certainly no grand theories to address the plight of the world's poor. But although *we* appear impotent to solve *their* problems, permitted a modest level of intellectual potential, in some spheres *they* just might.

Like others before him, the great philanthropist of Victorian England, Charles Booth, was clear about the dual approach that was needed to address the problems of the poor. 'There are two distinct tasks: to raise the general level of existence, but especially at the bottom, is one; to increase the proportion of those who know how to use aright the means they have is another.'[19] In the context of our current era, he could have been writing an EMID prevention policy, and it is interesting that he did not use the word 'education' to describe his second task. The fundamental strategy to increase the numbers of those who can 'use aright the means they have' is to *protect* those means – innate intellectual potential. It is no longer adequate just to educate intellects that have already declined because of environmentally mediated injuries.

But it is not just day-to-day existence that demands a functional level of intelligence across populations. This is also crucial for effective governance and justice. Alexis de Tocqueville put this point in a very straightforward manner in *Democracy in America*: 'legislators show little confidence in human honesty, but they always assume men are intelligent. So they generally rely on personal interest to see to the execution of the laws.'[20] Human well-being is certainly threatened by selfish interest, but it is very dependent on enlightened *self*-interest. And we require a functional level of intelligence to become enlightened, and to determine and assess what our interests are.

The positive survival of any human community now depends more on the ability of *all* levels of its population to act intelligently and adapt to change than on the number of PhD graduates it produces. The 1991 Club of Rome report, *The First Global Revolution*,[21] makes the broad argument, concluding that we can no longer rely on the genius of the few. Instead, 'thousands of small, wise decisions reflecting the new realisation of millions of ordinary people, are necessary for securing the survival of society'. Wise decisions are more likely in communities in which intellectual potential is not significantly impaired. 'Think global, act local' is a fine maxim to promote environmentally friendly behaviour, but it assumes that people in the locality are *able* to think and act effectively. People cannot make good choices if they have difficulty understanding the options.

The security of intellectual resources must become an environmental priority. Human protection in countless other important spheres would then follow in the wake of this guiding policy, but protection of the brain does not follow so readily in the path of other environmental health concerns, such as cancer or respiratory ailments. Putting the human brain first could challenge many existing environmental priorities. Global warming, for example, may slip down the list because its impact is likely to be slow and relatively manageable. And there could even be benefits: a warmer climate could provide new access to unpolluted land in northern Russia, for example. With a few exceptions, global warming will increase existing health problems that do not pose a major threat to the brain when compared, for example, with the immanent threat from lead contamination or the new hormone-disrupting chemicals.[22]

Whether or not the security of intellectual resources constitutes a grand ideology, which conflicts with the postmodern thesis, is a peripheral discussion. In a world where the population might double in forty years, common sense suggests that we will all muddle through a bit better if the collective intelligence of that new mass of humanity is at least broadly functional. The present prognosis is that this may not be so.

But the most significant meaning we can derive from the evidence currently available is not about eco-intelligence or regressive brain evolution, the inevitable cost to governments, or even about increasing social divides. The main message is about people as individuals. And already, for too many, it is too late.

# Notes

1. Chapter 2, Scale of effect.

2. Chapter 3, Adverse synergism.

3. Chapter 6, Unbounded lessons.

4. Chapter 7, Iatrogenicity.

5. Chapter 10, From the ecosystem's perspective.

6. Chapter 9, The evolutionary context.

7. Chapter 9, Ecological mechanisms.

8. Chapter 2, Social costs and consequences.

9. Chapter 9, The evolutionary context. John C. Eccles, *Evolution of the Brain: Creation of the Self* (Routledge: London, 1989), p. 224.

10. Chapter 10, The uniqueness of the human intellect.

11. Chapter 10, Pertinacity.

12. Chapter 10, The intellect in the ecosystem.

13. Francis Crick, *The Astonishing Hypothesis* (Touchstone Books: London, 1994), p. 256.

14. 'Algae for kingdom' (Report of a conference paper given by David Williams of the Natural History Museum in London), *Times Higher Education Supplement*, 13 September 1996, p. 6.

15. Chapter 10, From the ecosystem's perspective.

16. N.J. Mackintosh, 'Intelligence and reasoning', in T.W. Robbins and P. J. Cooper (eds), *Psychology for Medicine* (Edward Arnold: London, 1988), p. 135. J.R. Flynn, 'The mean IQ of Americans: massive gains 1932 to 1978', *Psychological Bulletin* (1984), **95**, 29–51. J. Flynn, 'Massive IQ gains in 14 nations: what IQ tests really measure', *Psychological Bulletin* (1987), **101**, 171–91. P.W. Fuggle *et al.*, 'Rising IQ scores in British children: recent evidence', *Journal of Child Psychology and Psychiatry* (1992), **33**, 1241–8.

17. Chapter 2, Personal costs and consequences.

18. Chapter 8, Education.

19. Charles Booth, *Life and Labour of the People in London* (Macmillan: London, 1902), p. 201.

20. Alexis de Tocqueville, *Democracy in America*, Vol.1 (Harper & Row: New York, 1966), p. 96 (first published 1835).

21. Alexander King and Bertrand Schneider, *The First Global Revolution: A Report by the Council of the Club of Rome* (Simon & Schuster: London, 1991), p. 183.

22. See Appendix.

# The Erice Statement

This consensus statement was issued on 30 May 1996, by an international group of scientists and physicians, following a workshop held on 5–10 November 1995 at Erice, Italy.

Hormones are chemical messengers that travel in the blood stream, turning on and off critical bodily functions to maintain health and well being. Taken together, the tissues and organs that produce, and respond to, hormones are called the endocrine system. The *Erice Statement* focuses attention on industrial chemicals that can interfere with the development of the brain and other parts of the central nervous system.

## Background

Research since 1991 has reinforced concerns over the scope of the problems posed to human health and ecological systems by endocrine-disrupting chemicals. New evidence is especially worrisome because it underscores the exquisite sensitivity of the developing nervous system to chemical perturbations that result in functional abnormalities. Moreover, the consequences of these perturbations depend upon the stage of development during which exposure occurs and are expressed in different ways at different times in life, from birth through to advanced age. This work session was conceived because of the growing concern that failure to confront the problem could have major economic and societal implications.

## Consensus statement

### 1. We are certain of the following:

Endocrine-disrupting chemicals can undermine neurological and behavioural development and subsequent potential of individuals exposed in the womb or, in fish, amphibians, reptiles, and birds, the egg. This loss of potential in humans and wildlife is expressed in behavioural and physical abnormalities. It may be expressed as reduced intellectual capacity and social adaptability, as impaired responsiveness to environmental demands, or in a variety of other functional guises. Widespread loss of this in nature can change the character of human societies or destabilize wildlife populations. Because profound economic and social consequences emerge from small shifts in functional potential at the population level, it is imperative to monitor levels of contaminants in humans, animals, and the environment that are associated with disruption of the nervous and endocrine systems and reduce their production and release.

Because the endocrine system is sensitive to perturbation, it is a likely target for disturbance. In contrast to natural hormones found in animals and plants, some of the components and by-products of many manufactured organic compounds that interfere with the endocrine system are persistent and undergo biomagnification in the food web, which makes them of greater concern as endocrine disruptors.

Man-made endocrine-disrupting chemicals range across all continents and oceans. They are found in native populations from the Arctic to the tropics, and, because of their persistence in the body, can be passed from generation to generation. The seriousness of the problem is exacerbated by the extremely low levels of hormones produced naturally by the endocrine system which are needed to modulate and induce appropriate responses. In contrast, many endocrine-disrupting contaminants, even if less potent than the natural products, are presented in living tissue at concentrations millions of times higher than the natural hormones. Wildlife, laboratory animals, and humans exhibit adverse health effects at contemporary environmental concentrations of man-made chemicals that act as endocrine disruptors. New technology has revealed that some man-made chemicals are present in tissue at concentrations previously not possible to measure with conventional analytical methods, but at concentrations which are biologically active.

Gestational exposure to persistent man-made chemicals reflects the lifetime exposure of females before they become pregnant. Hence, the transfer of contaminants to the developing embryo and foetus during pregnancy and to the newborn during lactation is not simply a function of recent maternal exposure. For some egg-laying species, the body burden of the females just prior to ovulation is the most critical period. For mammals, exposure to endocrine disruptors occurs during all of prenatal and early postnatal development because they are stored in the mother.

The developing brain exhibits specific and often narrow windows during which exposure to endocrine disruptors can produce permanent changes in its structure and function. The timing of exposure is crucial during early developmental stages, particularly during fetal development when a fixed sequence of structural change is occurring and before protective mechanisms have developed. A variety of chemical challenges in humans and animals early in life can lead to profound and irreversible abnormalities in brain development at exposure levels that do not produce permanent effects in adults.

Thyroid hormones are essential for normal brain functions through life. Interference with thyroid function during development leads to abnormalities in brain and behavioural development. The eventual results of moderate to severe alterations of thyroid hormone concentrations, particularly during fetal life, are motor dysfunction of varying severity including cerebral palsy, mental retardation, learning disability, attention deficit hyperactivity disorder, hydrocephalus, seizures and other permanent neurological abnormalities. Similarly, exposure to man-made chemicals during early development can impair motor function, spatial perception, learning, memory, auditory development, fine motor coordination, balance, and attentional processes; in severe cases, mental retardation may result.

Sexual development of the brain is under the influence of estrogenic (female) and androgenic (male) hormones. Not all endocrine disruptors are estrogenic or anti-estrogenic. For example, new data reveal that DDE, a breakdown product of DDT, found in almost all living tissue, is an anti-androgen in mammals. Man-made chemicals that interfere with sex hormones will have the potential to disturb normal brain sexual development. Wildlife studies of gulls, terns, fishes, whales, porpoises, alligators, and turtles link environmental contaminants with disturbances in sex hormone production and/or action. These effects have been associated with exposure to sewage and industrial effluents, pesticides, ambient ocean and freshwater contamination, and the aquatic food web.

Commonalities across species in the hormonal mechanisms controlling brain development and function mean that adverse effects observed in wildlife and laboratory animals may also occur in humans, although specific effects may differ from species to species. Most important, the same man-made chemicals that have shown these effects in mechanistic studies in laboratory animals also have a high exposure potential for humans.

The full range of substances interfering with natural endocrine modulations of neural and behavioural development cannot be entirely defined at present. However, compounds shown to have endocrine effects include dioxins, PCBs, phenolics, phthalates, and many pesticides. Any compounds mimicking or antagonizing actions of, or altering levels of, neurotransmitters, hormones, and growth factors in the developing brain are potentially in this group.

## 2.  We estimate with confidence that:

Every pregnant woman in the world has endocrine disruptors in her body that are transferred to the foetus. She also has measurable concentrations of endocrine disruptors in her milk that are transferred to the infant.

There may not be definable thresholds for responses to endocrine disruptors. In addition, for naturally occurring hormones, too much can be as severe a problem as too little. Consequently, simple (monotonic) dose–response curves for toxicity do not necessarily apply to the effects of endocrine disruptors.

Because certain PCBs and dioxins are known to impair normal thyroid function, we suspect that they contribute to learning disabilities, including attention deficit hyperactivity disorder and perhaps other neurological abnormalities. In addition, many pesticides affect thyroid function and, therefore, may have similar consequences.

Some endocrine disruptors or their breakdown products are nearly equipotent to [i.e. as powerful as] natural hormones. Even weak endocrine disruptors may exert potent effects because they can bypass the natural protection of blood binding proteins for endogenous [natural] hormones. Some disruptors also have a substantially longer biological half-life than naturally produced hormones because they are not readily metabolized, and as a result are stored in the body and accumulate to concentrations of concern. Some man-made chemicals that appear non-toxic are converted by the liver to more toxic compounds. Also, compounds that are not toxic in the mother may be toxic to her developing embryo, foetus or newborn. The exquisite vulnerability of the fetal brain to methylmercury and lead are prime examples of this principle.

Functional deficits are not as easily measured as physical anomalies or clinical disease, in part because they are typically expressed as continuous measures, such as IQ, rather than the number of cases in a population. Consequently, conventional population surveys may overlook the extent of such deficits. Moreover, because such surveys tend to express their findings as shifts in mean [average] values even when they are based on appropriate measures, they tend to obscure influences on the more susceptible members of the population.

Large amounts of man-made chemicals capable of disrupting the endocrine and nervous systems are sold to, or produced and used in, third world countries that lack the resources or technology to properly monitor and control exposure levels. Insufficient and improper training in handling chemicals and ignorance concerning health effects and monitoring strategies lead to the likelihood of very high levels of exposure.

## 3.   There are many uncertainties in our understanding because:

No one is exposure-free, thus confounding studies to determine what is normal. Everyone is exposed at any single time and throughout life to large numbers of man-made chemicals. Relatively few of the man-made chemicals found in human tissue have been identified. Lack of funding has seriously constrained testing these chemicals for their potential to disrupt natural systems.

Sensitive parameters, including neurological abnormalities, behavioural and neuropsychiatric disorders, and neuroanatomical, neurochemical, and neurophysiologic endpoints need to be investigated. Most important, criteria at the population level need to include the social and economic costs of impairment because the true costs to society of such problems can be significant, e.g. the costs of a 5 point IQ loss across a population. Investigation of potential toxicity typically includes laboratory, population and field studies, clinical reports, and accident reports. However, developmental neurotoxicants produce a spectrum of effects that are not typically evaluated, such as the progression and latency of behavioural and neurological changes. In addition, alteration of other systems can produce subsequent cognitive, behavioural, and neurological dysfunction; i.e. diseases of other organ systems that influence the brain; non-CNS [central nervous system] drugs; other foreign substances such as air pollutants; and immune system involvements that alter behaviour.

Trade secret laws afford industry confidentiality, depriving the consumer and public health authorities of the right to know the components of commercial products so they can be tested.

## 4.   Our judgment is that:

The benefits of reduced health care costs could be substantial if exposure to endocrine-disrupting chemicals were reduced.

A trivial amount of governmental resources is devoted to monitoring environmental chemicals and health effects. The public are unaware of this and believe that they are adequately protected. The message that endocrine disruptors are present in the environment and have the potential to affect many people over a lifespan has not effectively reached the general public, the scientific community, regulators, or policy makers. Although this message is difficult to reduce to simple statements without over- or under-stating the problem, the potential risks to human health are so widespread and far-reaching that any policy based on continued ignorance of the facts would be unconscionable.

The outcome of exposure is inadequately addressed when based just on population averages. Instead, risk should be based on the range of responses within a population – that is, the total distribution. The magnitude of the problem can be better determined by knowing the distribution of responses to endocrine disruptors by individuals within subsets of the population most at risk, such as pregnant women, developing embryos, foetuses, and newborns, teens, the aged, the ill or those with pre-existing endocrine disorders. The magnitude of the risks also depends upon the endpoint [i.e. health effect] under consideration. For example, a variety of motor, sensory, behavioural, and cognitive functions, endpoints which are more sensitive than cancer, must be considered when assessing neurological function. This holds for wildlife and domestic animals, as well as human populations.

Wildlife have been effective models for understanding endocrine disruption at the molecular, cellular, individual, population, and ecosystem levels. Future research to examine diverse wildlife species at all levels of biological organization must be broadened and adequately supported.

Those responsible for producing man-made chemicals must assure product safety beyond a reasonable doubt. Manufacturers should be required to release the names of all chemicals used in their products with the appropriate evidence that the products pose no developmental health hazard.

Current panels of scientists who determine the distribution of public research funds often have a narrow scope of expertise and are thus ill-equipped to review the kind of interdisciplinary research that is necessary in this field. Funding institutions should be encouraged to increase the scope of representation on review panels and to develop more appropriate mechanisms for interdisciplinary reviews. Governmental agencies should also increase funding for multidisciplinary extramural projects for surveillance of wildlife and human populations where neurological damage is suspected and follow any leads with laboratory research. In addition, populations of animals consuming the contaminated foods also eaten by humans should be studied for developmental health effects. It is important to observe a variety of vertebrate species through multigenerational studies.

Strategies for increasing interdisciplinary communication and collaborations to optimize resources and future research are needed. Studies should be designed more economically to include the sharing of material among many collaborators. Interdisciplinary teams should explore neurological and other types of damage at all levels of biological organization from molecular through biochemical, physiological, and behavioural.

A concerted effort should be undertaken to deliver this consensus statement to the public, key decision makers, and the media. In addition, specially designed messages should be developed for family physicians and others responsible for public health who are often unaware of the possible role of occupational and environmental chemical pollutants as agents underlying or constituting risk factors for 'primary' human diseases. Physicians must be trained in medical school about often latent effects of pollutants on human development and health. This training is currently inadequate. A coordinated speakers bureau and on-line systems such as a site on the World Wide Web for endocrine disruptors should be established.

Reproduced with thanks from *Rachel's Environment & Health Weekly*, nos. 263 and 264.

Environmental Research Foundation, PO Box 5036, Annapolis, MD 21403-7036, USA.

# Sources of Further Information

*Environmentally-Mediated Intellectual Decline (EMID): A Selected Interdisciplinary Bibliography*, Dr Christopher Williams, includes the documents used in *Terminus Brain*, and other relevant sources of information. It is available from:

The Administrator
The Global Security Programme
University of Cambridge
Botolph House
17 Botolph Lane
Cambridge CB2 3RE
UK

or

The Administrator
Education and International Development
Institute of Education
University of London
20 Bedford Way
London WC1H 0AL
UK

# Index